GOOD SPORT

To Barbara and Mark

May your years be
filled with good sport.

Warmest best wishes,

Tim

April 2019

GOOD SPORT

Why Our Games Matter—And How Doping
Undermines Them

Thomas H. Murray

OXFORD
UNIVERSITY PRESS

OXFORD
UNIVERSITY PRESS

Oxford University Press is a department of the University of Oxford. It furthers
the University's objective of excellence in research, scholarship, and education
by publishing worldwide. Oxford is a registered trade mark of Oxford University
Press in the UK and certain other countries.

Published in the United States of America by Oxford University Press
198 Madison Avenue, New York, NY 10016, United States of America.

Library of Congress Cataloging-in-Publication Data
Names: Murray, Thomas H., 1946– author.
Title: Good sport : why our games matter—and how doping undermines them /
by Thomas H. Murray.
Description: New York, NY : Oxford University Press, [2018] |
Includes bibliographical references.
Identifiers: LCCN 2017005059 | ISBN 9780190687984 (hardback) |
ISBN 9780190687991 (Updf)
Subjects: LCSH: Doping in sports—Moral and ethical aspects. | Athletes—Drug
use—Moral and ethical aspects. | BISAC: SPORTS & RECREATION /
Sociology of Sports. | SPORTS & RECREATION / General. | PHILOSOPHY /
Ethics & Moral Philosophy.
Classification: LCC RC1230 .M87 2017 | DDC 362.29088/796—dc23
LC record available at https://lccn.loc.gov/2017005059

1 3 5 7 9 8 6 4 2

Printed by Sheridan Books, Inc., United States of America

To my beloved grandchildren, Grace, Tess, Cooper and Alice.
May you find great joy, challenge, and fulfillment in sport
and in your lives

CONTENTS

ACKNOWLEDGMENTS

When a book takes as many years to write as this one, it's impossible to recognize, or even remember, every person whose thoughts or help went into its creation. Some names, however, stand out. Thanks first of all to the Hastings Center research assistants who helped me sift through the massive literature on sport as it touched on doping, gender, technology in sport, health risks, and the Paralympics: Colleen Farrell, Polo Black Golde, Alison Jost, Jacob Moses, Cameron Waldman, and Ross White. Thanks likewise to Michelle Bayefsky and Alissa Wassung, students at Yale who were so helpful in identifying important sources. Thanks also to members of the extended Hastings family for their unflagging encouragement and faith in the project, among them Mary Crowley, Michael Patterson, David Roscoe, and Frank Trainer. No list would be complete without mentioning Jodi Fernandes who, as Assistant to the President of the Center, helped keep me sane and grounded in the midst of the all-too-frequent crises prone to erupt at a small, fiercely independent, and far from wealthy ethics research institute. Many thanks to the World Anti-Doping Agency for the 2009 grant to The Hastings Center that allowed me to begin work on this book. Without that support freeing up a portion of my time to devote to this project, responsible as I was for the Center's well being, it would have been years before any progress would have been possible.

I've learned so much from athletes, anti-doping pioneers, and others devoted to values and meanings in sport. Among those who generously shared their insights with me are Alison Carlson, Dave Ellis, Myron Genel, David Gerrard, Doug Glanville, Mike McNamee, Aimee Mullins, Bill Peace, and David Weisbrot. I am especially grateful to my long-time colleagues and friends in the movement to preserve a place for clean sport: Jim Betts, Don Catlin, and Edwin Moses.

As the book took final shape, many experts read substantial portions of the manuscript and offered helpful comments and corrections including Stéphane Bermon, Larry Bowers, Rob Donovan, Martha Farah, Gary Green, Joanna Harper, John Hoberman, David Howman, Greg Kaebnick, Rob Koehler, Arne Ljungqvist, Sigmund Loland, María José Martínez Patiño, Jamie Nelson, Martin Ritzen, Peter Van De Vliet and Eric Vilain. In addition I am blessed with friends on Cape Cod including Brian and Joan Condon, Paul and Peggy Kelleher, and Pat and Eduardo Marti, whose insights and (in Eduardo's case) translations from Spanish into English are reflected in the book. Peter Ohlin, my editor at OUP, was unfailingly supportive and improved the final text with his insightful suggestions.

None of this would have been possible or worth doing without the love of my family: my wife and partner in life, Cynthia, my children and grandchildren Kate, Nicky, Andie, Grace, Tess, Cooper and Alice. A very special thanks to my son Pete Murray for his invaluable help thinking through the relevance for sport of John Rawls's writings on justice. And to my son-in-law, Matt Rennie, sports editor extraordinaire, for his exceptionally helpful and thorough comments on the entire draft of the book.

Neither of my parents lived to see the publication of this book, yet they each deserve heartfelt thanks for whatever merit it may have. My father was an avid baseball fan and a mostly patient teacher. The times he took me to see his beloved Phillies play were highlights of the summer. Watching him chase my errant throws into the street when we played catch, less so. He taught me to persevere and to find satisfaction, even occasional joy, in the pursuit of excellence. My mother encouraged me to aim high. When my book *The Worth of a Child* was published she wanted to know why I hadn't written a best seller. They loved me, I knew it, and, even if I didn't become the doctor they'd envisioned, they took pride in whatever I was able to accomplish.

Finally, to Cynthia's and my beloved daughter Emily. Where others found joy participating in sports, she loved theatre, singing, and dancing. We miss her presence, but we are profoundly grateful for the time we shared with her.

INTRODUCTION

Around 1980 I began conversations with athletes and others involved in Olympic and professional sport. I asked them, in effect, two questions: Why does any athlete use performance-enhancing drugs? Why does it matter whether doping affects the outcome of competitions?

My decades-long journey to understand the ethics of performance-enhancing drug use in sport turned up other persistent questions. Sport accepts many technologies that boost athletes' performances such as fiberglass poles and hinged skates—why ban drugs? Why do we prohibit certain drugs but permit sophisticated nutritional supplements? Athletes are sometimes allowed to use otherwise prohibited drugs under a so-called therapeutic use exemption. How are those exemptions granted and what justifies them?

Look more closely, though, and you will find that sport has an ambivalent relationship with technologies that improve performance. Swimming banned impermeable full-body suits swimmers wore to smash records. Golf barred balls that fly straighter and clubs that diminish the cost of hitting into the rough. This refusal to make things easier is a vital clue pointing to the core values that bind together all sports: respect for natural talents, the perseverance and dedication required to perfect those talents, and the courage to risk failure when lining up against comparably talented competitors.

These values explain how sport responds to innovations in strategies and equipment. They provide the framework for understanding sport's commitment to creating "level playing fields." Meaningful and interesting competitions in which talent and dedication are the most important factors shaping outcomes rather than age, size, gender, or superior equipment are meant to reward talent, dedication, and courage. The same values permeate the Paralympics. In addition to the other factors shaping outcomes, Paralympic competitions also have to take into account the particular type of impairment as well as its severity.

The answer to my first question—why do athletes ever use drugs—made it clear that athletes feel enormous pressure *not* to surrender an edge to their drug-using competitors. Doping sets in motion a relentless competitive dynamic capable of pushing drug use to epidemic levels. The world saw the dynamic's corrosive impact in the Lance Armstrong era in bike racing.

It took me many years to answer the second question. Decades of wrestling with difficult questions working with the U.S. Olympic Committee, chairing the Ethics Panel for the World Anti-Doping Agency, and now as a member of the International Association of Athletics Federations' Independent Ethics Board provided abundant opportunities to learn and to test out ideas. Protecting athletes' health, of course, was an important part of the answer. But doping doesn't have to be dangerous to corrupt sport. It's enough that doping undermines what gives sport its value and meaning. Sport's devotion to natural talents, dedication, and courage answers my second question. Performance-enhancing drugs distort the connection between natural talents, the dedication to perfect those talents, and success in sport. That's good enough reason to ban doping.

Even with a firm commitment to the value of drug-free sport, questions remain. How best can we protect athletes' health? Can anti-doping be effective in the face of powerful incentives to dope and the complicity of scientists, physicians, coaches and, at times, nation states? Is the effort to limit doping's impact on sport worth the trouble and expense? What must sport do to assure its integrity and to free itself of corruption?

Finally, what's at stake in the future when an ideal of sport that values natural talents, dedication, and courage encounters would-be competitors with technologically enhanced bodies far beyond anything possible today?

Good Sport illuminates how rejecting doping doesn't hold competitors to an arbitrary standard but rather preserves and uplifts the values that give sport its meaning.

Chapter 1

The Slippery Slope to Doping

That was when I decided I didn't want to be a pro cyclist any
more. I got home and decided: 'No, thank you'. I love cycling,
it's a beautiful sport, but it would have been very difficult
for me to look anyone in the eye and say I was clean when
I wasn't.

Scott Mercier

Tyler Hamilton won Olympic Gold in the 2004 bicycling time
trial, a brutal all-out race against the clock. Hamilton's victory
came after three years on the U.S. Postal Service team helping
Lance Armstrong take home the victor's yellow jersey in the grueling three-week endurance test that is the Tour de France. Lithe
but powerful, Hamilton specialized in wearing out Armstrong's
rivals as they labored up the Col du Tourmalet, Mont Ventoux,
and other steep climbs.

Like his teammate Armstrong and fellow American Floyd
Landis, who won the Tour in 2006, Hamilton was on drugs. Each
year, the Tour's top three finishers stand on a podium to receive
their prizes. Of the thirty riders who stood on that podium from
1998 through 2007, at least twenty-two have either confessed or
been officially linked to using performance-enhancing drugs.

We know Hamilton was using performance-enhancing drugs
because, after repeated denials, he confessed the details in his
2012 memoir *The Secret Race*. The book is a well of sadness; still,
what I found most revealing was his story of the little white bag.[1]

When he began riding with the Postal Service team, Hamilton first noticed the lunch-bag-size sacks, folded neatly at the top. A pattern was clear: They were given only to the most successful riders. He heard other riders boast (if they rode well) or lament (if they didn't), that they were "riding paniagua." Eventually, he figured out they were saying *"pan y agua"*—Spanish for "bread and water"—team lingo for racing without the aid of drugs. Riding well without doping was uncommon enough to deserve mention. Hamilton initially loathed the white bags, becoming fixated on them. Then he was invited to become a member of the white bag club. He had proven himself; he had joined the elite.

Soon, Hamilton was doping like a winner. When EPO—a hormone that boosts endurance—reigned, bike racers were convinced they had to dope because the drugs made you so much faster—five to seven percent according to some estimates. Add to that the widely held belief that many other riders were doping: Under those circumstances, riding clean was equivalent to unilateral disarmament in war—basically, conceding defeat. For an ambitious young rider such as Hamilton, the power of performance-enhancing drugs was understood before exposure to European professional bike racing. But Hamilton could not anticipate how deeply interwoven and casually accepted doping was in that culture.

My first glimpse into the forces shaping athletes' choices began around 1980, twenty-four years before Tyler Hamilton's tainted Olympic triumph. As part of a research project into drug use outside of treating illness, I spoke with elite athletes and their coaches, scientists and doctors, and, later, people involved in anti-doping—the effort to keep artificial enhancements out of sport. What I found was, in roughly equal measure, startling and disheartening. In sports where anabolic steroids or stimulants made a discernible difference, doping was rampant. I wondered why, so I asked the athletes. Their answers were remarkably consistent, perceptive, and glum.

I was told then—and many, many times since—the usual reason athletes decide to dope is their belief that their competition already is doing so—and no one wants to lose, especially to an ostensibly inferior foe. Any athlete who achieves elite status does so through talent and dedication. In this select company, though, everyone has extraordinary gifts, and everyone labors to perfect them. So pretty much the only way to have a shot at winning is to match any edge the opponent seeks. Performance-enhancing drugs provide a competitive advantage too great to overcome.

Jonathan Vaughters, another of Lance Armstrong's teammates, described the choice a talented, ambitious young cyclist faced in an era when doping was endemic: "Almost every athlete I've met who has doped will say they did it only because they wanted a level playing field. That says something: everyone wants a fair chance, not more. Young cyclists' identities were intimately tied up with success in their sport. In many instances they had foregone other life opportunities to concentrate on this one avenue."[2]

Like Tyler Hamilton, David Millar, another prominent bike racer, saw a culture that seemed to violate what he and other athletes loved about cycling in the first place. Millar told an interviewer: "It got to a point where it was almost easier for me to dope than not to," he said, pain clouding his face. "Psychologically I just gave in, I couldn't fight it any more, it seemed like such a lost cause. No one seemed to care: not the team bosses or heads of the sport. Even the media seemed naive and blind to it all. So many things built to that point. It was an accumulation of little things, a deterioration of character and my ethical standards."[3]

There were two other unhappy options: compete without drugs, and face almost inevitable defeat, even to those less talented and dedicated; or give up competing at the highest level, despite having the necessary talent and discipline. Bike racing offers examples of both.

Bradley Mcgee, Australian Olympic track cyclist and Tour de France competitor refused to dope and paid the price: "I was competing not just against Armstrong, but against the Armstrong years. I feel my professional years—my Tour de France years— have been stolen . . . The more I think about it, the more it makes me mad as hell. But I have to move on from the fact that I have, more than likely, missed out on results and revenue, plus more, because of others' doping."[4]

Scott Mercier didn't want to dope, and wasn't reconciled to losing or lying. In May 1997 he was summoned to the U.S. Postal team physician's hotel room: "[the physician] handed me a bag containing a bottle of green pills and several vials of clear liquid . . . I was given a 17-day training schedule too. Each day had either a dot or a star. A dot represented a pill and a star was an injection. He said: 'They're steroids, you go strong like bull.' Then he said: 'Put it in your pocket, if you get stopped at customs say it's B vitamins.' That was when I decided I didn't want to be a pro cyclist any more. I got home and decided: 'No, thank you'. I love cycling, it's a beautiful sport, but it would have been very difficult for me to look anyone in the eye and say I was clean when I wasn't."[5]

ANTI-DOPING TO GIVE CLEAN ATHLETES A FAIR CHANCE

Anti-doping programs seek to create a fourth and better option: providing a competitive environment free from artificial performance enhancement where you win or lose based on how talented and disciplined you are. An environment in which the

Bradley McGees of the world wouldn't miss out on the rewards they deserved; where the Scott Merciers wouldn't have to walk away from their dreams. And where the Tyler Hamiltons and David Millars wouldn't have believed that doping was their only possible path to success.

It's not just cycling. In any sport where doped athletes have notable advantages, all athletes feel the effects. Doug Glanville was a very successful Major League Baseball player with a 200-hit season—a remarkable accomplishment. Glanville played in the steroids era. He's wondered whether his career was shortened because he had to compete for a roster spot against bulked-up outfielders hitting more home runs than he ever could without using muscle-building drugs.[6] Swimming, wrestling, weightlifting, sprinting short distances, running long ones, throwing hammers, shotputs, or discuses—name the sport, and if doping can enhance someone's performance, someone's tried it. And you can bet that other athletes in that sport suspected it and faced the same doleful choices.

It took sport decades to get serious about creating that fourth option: competition that offers reasonable confidence that the winners aren't doping. The challenges are daunting: a pipeline endlessly supplying new ways to dope; the difficulty of maintaining a complicated system for deterring and detecting doped athletes and corrupt coaches, trainers, doctors, and officials; and athletes eager to win but, even more, unwilling to lose to someone who's chemically enhanced.

Reliable numbers are hard to come by, and people throw out attention-grabbing, unverifiable figures for the percentage of competitors doping in one sport or another. On occasion, the walls of secrecy crumble, and we get a glimpse of the ruins within. East Germany dominated women's swimming in the 1970s not because their athletes were more gifted or worked harder, but because they had created a ruthless doping machine with more than one hundred scientists and physicians experimenting with the health of countless young athletes. When American swimmer Shirley Babashoff called attention to the masculine bodies and deep voices of the German swimmers at the 1976 Montreal Summer Olympics, the German coach responded dismissively, "We have come to swim, not to sing."[7] Indeed, they swam very well. And many paid a heavy price later from the powerful hormones pumped into their bodies.[8]

The process of letting daylight into bike racing was dramatically punctuated with the U.S. Anti-Doping Agency's "reasoned decision" that exposed Lance Armstrong's bullying and lies.[9] I've spoken with leaders of that investigation who describe cyclists' relief and catharsis once they unburdened themselves of the toxic secrets they'd hidden for years. The pro cyclists I've met who'd spoken with USADA investigators confirm that impression. Were they sincere? The cynical view is the witnesses were contrite in hopes of receiving reduced sanctions for their own misdeeds, a more forgiving public reception, or both. But the other interpretation is that they genuinely felt they'd done something wrong. If indeed they felt guilty about doping, two possibilities remain: either there really is something fundamentally wrong with doping in sport; or as some claim, doping is perfectly okay but athletes, like most people, are just confused about the ethics of doping.

HEALTH RISKS, PATERNALISM, AND THE ETHICS OF ANTI-DOPING

Norman Fost, one of the early critics of anti-doping, thinks the confusion starts with the risks of doping. Back in 1986, Fost pointed to the lack of conclusive scientific evidence on doping's dangers to health.[10] He was right that the dire warnings broadcast by "experts" at that time were based on scant data, more designed to frighten athletes than to inform them. But there were plausible reasons for concern when athletes were taking massively more of these potent hormones than the amounts recommended for therapy: twenty times the dose twice a week rather than a much smaller amount every three or four weeks, according to the evidence I saw. And they didn't stop with just one drug: They would stack multiple drugs in bespoke combinations so drug-on-drug interactions were also a source of worry.

Our ignorance at that time had many causes. Doping lived in the shadows; athletes were reluctant to admit it, and it's hard to study what you can't see. The drugs athletes thought they were using often came from illicit sources, making it difficult to know what the real compounds and dosages were, a problem that continues today with many supplements. (Terry Todd, a champion powerlifter, told the story of finding an ad for "gorilla growth hormone." Making even a tiny quantity of actual gorilla growth hormone would require an implausible number of gorilla pituitary glands. Todd bought some and had it analyzed. Indeed, there was no gorilla or growth hormone in the mix. Still, the prospect of injections that would give you the strength of a gorilla may have been enough for some gullible customers.) Money to do the research was almost nonexistent. And the committees entrusted with protecting people by balancing the risks of research against the hoped-for benefits would have a devil of a time justifying an experiment that gave massive doses of powerful drugs to healthy young people just to see what damage was done. The risks were potentially grave; the benefits, elusive.

For Fost and some other critics, the health risks of doping don't really matter. Even if the risks are significant, Fost complained that preventing athletes from doping is a form of paternalism—philosophical shorthand for making decisions for another person without regard for how that individual weighs the risks and benefits. "Whether or not a competent person seeks pleasure or financial gain involving risk is a personal decision. So long as the activity is not imposing burdens involuntarily on others, we reject paternalistic interference with risky behavior."[10 (p6-7)] People don't like to be told what to do, especially under the premise that it's for their own good. Fans of the movie *A Christmas Story* will recall the paternalistic reason every adult gave Ralphie for why he shouldn't get a Red Rider BB gun as a gift: "You'll shoot your eye out!" (His father gave him one anyway.)

Fost's article was in response to one I had published three years earlier in which I described the great pressures athletes experienced to use performance-enhancing drugs in order to remain competitive. From what athletes had told me, those forces were so powerful many concluded they had no real choice but to comply. I dubbed what I'd observed the "coercive power" of drugs in sport. Fost was not persuaded. He distinguished between an offer and a threat. A threat is coercive and therefore an affront to individual liberty. But to him, the situation faced by athletes, including young athletes, was merely an offer. I believed then, and I believe now, that this view fails to understand how choices like these appear to aspiring young athletes. It also trivializes the intense pressures put on them from coaches, trainers, teammates, or sponsors to dope. The stories told by Tyler Hamilton, David Millar, Bradley McGee, Scott Mercier, and countless others make clear what's at stake when young athletes confront the choices doping forces upon them. You don't need to have a gun pointed at your head to feel like your future and your place in the world is at risk.

Fost had one more interesting objection to anti-doping: that the lines we draw between the unobjectionable stuff people put into their bodies such as food, vitamins, and supplements on the one hand and performance-enhancing drugs on the other are too fuzzy to justify banning the latter and not the former. And, he argued, because we wouldn't consider banning food, vitamins, or most supplements, we shouldn't ban drugs either. Of course sport draws lines regularly, such as every time it establishes the dimensions of a playing field, court, or goal. Understanding the criteria sport uses to determine dimensions, new equipment, and rules of play will help illuminate its response to artificial enhancements.

THE CRITICISMS MULTIPLY

Many anti-doping critics offer a multitude of reasons to radically redo or even abandon efforts to give athletes a chance to succeed without resorting to drugs. Some pick out practical imperfections in the current system, of which there are many: drugs we can't identify with today's tests; cheaters who escape detection; the striking incursions on athletes' privacy when we insist that they reveal where they are every day and that someone be watching when they pee into a sample jar.

Then there are conceptual puzzles. How can we justify banning EPO when there are other methods for enhancing endurance that we profess to have no problem with, such as training at altitude or using the strategy "train low/rest high" that requires spending much of the day and night in an artificial low-oxygen environment?

Finally come challenges to the very idea of what should constitute excellence in sport. Malcolm Gladwell defended Lance

Armstrong in a 2013 *New Yorker* article, "Man and Superman." He portrays Armstrong's doping as "a vision of sports in which the object of competition is to use science, intelligence, and sheer will to conquer natural difference."[11] Science, for Gladwell, includes the savvy use of drugs such as EPO, steroids, and human growth hormone. For him, natural differences in athletic abilities are obstacles to be overcome rather than talents to be honed and perfected. In Gladwell's view, doping is not merely tolerable in sport, but instead an essential tool for leveling the playing field. I believe he and other commentators with similar views misunderstand what's valuable in sport and what sport means to those who play it or watch it more than casually.

We need to hear what the critics say, give them their due when they deserve it, and answer them decisively where they're mistaken. As in the response to Fost's complaint that athletes should have the liberty to decide for themselves whether to dope, the answers often will begin with a careful look into the realities of sport: at athletes' hopes and fears; at how a sport decides whether to welcome or to ban particular innovations, such as golf balls that fly straight no matter what; at the ways sporting events such as the Paralympics try to stage meaningful and interesting competitions.

Most discussions of doping in sport don't bother asking why it might be wrong; they just assume that it is. I believe it's vital to ask that question forthrightly. I also believe it will be more interesting and illuminating if we begin not with what's wrong with doping, but with what gives sport, at its best, meaning and value. Consider the case of an Olympian who won the genetic lottery for cross-country skiing.

NOTES

1. Coyle D, Hamilton T. *The Secret Race: Inside the Hidden World of the Tour de France: Doping, Cover-ups, and Winning at All Costs.* New York: Bantam; 2012.
2. Vaughters J. How to get doping out of sports. *NYTimes.com.* 2012 Aug 8. Available from: http://www.nytimes.com/2012/08/12/opinion/sunday/how-to-get-doping-out-of-sports.html.
3. Swarbrick S. Cyclist David Millar tells of his battle with drugs. *The Herald* (Scotland). 2011 Sept. Available from: http://www.heraldscotland.com/life_style/13041664.Cyclist_David_Millar_tells_of_his_battle_with_drugs/ (Accessed 2017 Mar 13).
4. McGee B. How dopers stole the best years of my career. *Sydney Morning Herald.* 2012 Oct 27. Available from: http://www.smh.com.au/sport/cycling/how-dopers-stole-the-best-years-of-my-career 20121026 28aif.html (Accessed 2016 Dec 28).
5. Austin S. I quit cycling because of the drugs. Now I am Lance Armstrong's best riding buddy. 2014 Jan 9. Available from: http://www.telegraph.co.uk/sport/othersports/cycling/10562181/I-quit-cycling-because-of-the-drugs.-Now-I-am-Lance-Armstrongs-best-riding-buddy.html (Accessed 2015 May 5).
6. Glanville D. Desperately seeking blank. *The Pennsylvania Gazette.* 2010 July/Aug. Available from: http://www.upenn.edu/gazette/0710/feature2_1.html.
7. Amdur N. Mounting drug use afflicts world sports. *The New York Times.* 1978 Nov 20. Available from: http://www.nytimes.com/1978/11/20/archives/mounting-drug-use-afflicts-world-sports-drug-epidemic-afflicts.html (Accessed 2016 July 26).
8. Franke WW, Berendonk B. Hormonal doping and androgenization of athletes: A secret program of the German Democratic Republic government. *Clin Chem.* 1997;43(7):1262–1279.
9. U.S. Anti-Doping Agency (USADA) (n.d.) U.S. Postal Service Pro Cycling Team Investigation. Available from: http://cyclinginvestigation.usada.org/ (Accessed 2013 Dec 16).
10. Fost N. Banning drugs in sports: A skeptical view. *The Hastings Center Report* 1986;16(4):5–10.
11. Gladwell M. Man and superman. *The New Yorker.* 2013 Sept 9. Available from: http://www.newyorker.com/magazine/2013/09/09/man-and-superman (Accessed 2016 Mar 7).

Chapter 2

What Sport Values

NATURAL TALENTS AND HOW WE PERFECT THEM

I was not successful as a ball player, as it was a game of skill.

Casey Stengel

Wolfgang Amadeus Mozart wrote his first compositions by age five and his first symphony at eight—a child prodigy by any measure. His innate talent was obvious to everyone, including his father, who abandoned his own efforts to compose music when he saw what his young son was able to accomplish. Like a world-class athlete, Mozart was born with uncommon natural talent. His operas, symphonies, concertos, and more are wonderful because he possessed an extraordinary gift for music, and because he dedicated himself to honing that gift. Most exceptional things in life—great performances and great creations—require both.

Like all natural gifts, differences in raw athletic talents are unearned, and that bothers some people. Some see Steph Curry's grace on the basketball court as somehow "unfair," in a way they wouldn't characterize Mozart's brilliance as a composer and performer or Georgia O'Keefe's ability to use color and visual metaphor. But each inherited a talent and then worked to perfect it. We don't need a precise accounting here of what percentage can be attributed to inherited capacities versus the arduous cultivation of those "unearned" talents. You need both. Acknowledging the significance of the "unearned" in no way detracts from our appreciation of what's been accomplished.

How can we know whether differences in natural talents are fair or unfair in sport? A little thought experiment may help. Suppose I challenge Lebron James to a game of one-on-one basketball. Suppose also that I've been training intensively for six months—working just as diligently as Lebron to hone my skills. He's still going to whip my ass. Completely. Resoundingly. Humiliatingly. At barely 5 feet 11 and 170 pounds, entering my 70s, and with arthritic knees attesting to a youth spent on cement and blacktop courts, I stand no chance of winning. I'll be lucky to get off a single shot that won't be blocked or take two dribbles in a row before the ball is stolen. The only way it might interest spectators would be as comic relief.

Isn't this unfair? I worked as hard as Lebron. He just happens to be much taller, stronger, faster, and quicker than I am. He's also more agile, leaps higher, with superior reaction time and better eyesight. He didn't "earn" these abilities, any more than Eero Mäntyranta "earned" an abundance of red blood cells. (More on this exceptional Finnish cross-country skier in a moment.) I could devote a year to relentless training while Lebron could take to his recliner, eat donuts, and watch sitcoms, and the result would be the same. He's vastly more talented at basketball than I've ever been. That is so UNFAIR.

This complaint is, of course, ludicrous. No law of biology or ethics demands that every talent be given out in equal measure to all persons, or that victory go only to the most dedicated worker. Differences in natural, inherited talents are inescapable, and in fact, a celebrated part of sport. When athletes talk of a "level playing field," they don't mean neutralizing all differences in natural abilities. (And for what it's worth, to be truly the best requires extraordinary dedication. LeBron works as hard as anyone to hone his skills. He's transformed himself into a more complete basketball player and a better teammate every year. His extraordinary natural talents for basketball combined with his relentless determination to perfect those talents are why he has reached levels few athletes ever will.)

People vary in their talents for the full range of activities that humans engage in. Some have talents for hospitality and friendship, while others don't. Some can dance; others are painfully inept like the character Elaine on *Seinfeld*. Some are musical; some can't carry a tune. Some folks are brilliant thinkers; others are not. And some have talents that give them an advantage in particular sports, while others lack those gifts. But the fact that we're different doesn't mean that those differences are morally unfair. The worldview here is topsy-turvy. Sport is a celebration of the wonderful variety of human talents, along with the dedication individuals bring to perfecting those talents. Sport is not a morality contest meant to reward only the most virtuous.

The specific talents that matter vary from sport to sport. The slender torso, narrow hips, and skinny legs of a marathon runner's body don't make a successful super-heavyweight lifter. And heaven help the stocky muscular lifter trying to compete in a marathon. In team sports, different positions call for different skills. In American football, wide receivers can weigh half as much as offensive linemen, but they need to be fast, elusive, have great hands and the courage to catch a pass knowing they're likely to get hit. The physical gifts that lead to victory in curling don't lend themselves to pole-vaulting success, but so what?

If you know a sport well, you have a pretty good idea about the sorts of natural talents it requires. On the other hand, you don't need to know much about a sport to understand the essential role dedication plays. Bill Bradley, a transcendent basketball star at Princeton, later Rhodes Scholar, essential cog in a New York Knicks championship team, and US Senator, was famous for his discipline. He worked relentlessly on his shot. From selected spots on the floor he would shoot until he made twenty-five in a row. If he missed the twenty-fourth, the count started over. His desire to become the best player he could be demanded unceasing effort: "Driven to excel by some deep, unsurveyed urge, I stayed out on that floor hour after hour, day after day, year after year. I played until my muscles stiffened and my arms ached. I persevered through blisters, contusions, and strained joints."[1]

In his book *Values of the Game*, Bradley explains how his dedication grew: "In my experience, the feeling of getting better came with hard work, and getting better made victory easier. Winning was fun, but so was the struggle to improve. That was one of the lessons you learned from the game: Basketball was a clear example of virtue rewarded." In what he describes as "a game of subtle felonies," Bradley found joy, imagination, and meaning.

Great athletes such as Bill Bradley demonstrate talent, the dedication to perfect that talent, and the courage to test themselves. Raw talent alone is rarely enough. Neither is diligent training if the talent just isn't there. The meaning and value we find in sport comes from our sense of wonder at the natural talents displayed, and our admiration for the dedication required to bring those talents to their highest expression.

Dedication and courage are valuable character traits in all spheres of human life. Our circumstances and upbringing helped shape our character, certainly, but virtues must be cultivated, practiced, refined. Because they require persistent effort and don't just happen to us, we find these traits admirable, and we give people credit when we see them in action.

Natural talents, on the other hand, *do* just happen. We can choose whether or not to hone them, but we have no control over whether we have them or not. We can marvel at someone's inherited talents, but no one "deserves" or "earns" their raw talents, so those abilities aren't morally admirable in the same way that dedication and courage are. And there is no guarantee that whatever natural talents we inherit will be useful in any arena beyond their specific application. Mozart likely couldn't play basketball any better than LeBron James could compose music.

EERO MÄNTYRANTA'S GENETIC EDGE

Some commentators argue that this difference between our natural talents and the commendable things we do to perfect those talents should influence how we think about doping and genetic enhancement. Consider a case of a man born with an extraordinary talent: Eero Mäntyranta, Finnish cross-country skier and reindeer herder. Mäntyranta won two gold medals at the 1964 Winter Olympics in Innsbruck, Austria, seven Olympic medals overall. He also had a genetic abnormality known as inherited polycythemia that resulted in an unusually high concentration of red blood cells circulating in his body.[2] More red cells mean more oxygen for starving muscles and, thus, the capacity to carry on longer with physically taxing activities such as Nordic skiing.

Think of each of the roughly 20,000 genes in our body as a sentence—the smallest unit of meaning in the genetic language. Genomic sentences are prone to Faulknerian length: the gene responsible for Mäntyranta's extraordinary endurance is more than 500 words long. Unlike English, the genetic alphabet has just four letters: A, T, C and G. Every word in the genomic language is precisely three letters long. The language also has punctuation. Periods that signal "stop reading," are, like words, three letters in length.

Mäntyranta inherited a fascinating misspelling: The letter G was swapped out for an A in the 439th word of the genomic sentence instructing his cells to make a protein known as EPOR. The "R" in EPOR stands for "receptor." The normal EPOR protein helps our cells dance a graceful ballet. When it senses that there's plenty of EPO around, it announces, "Time to make more red blood cells!" When EPO is scarce, it shuts down production. Mäntyranta's version of the gene was missing the shutdown command. Changing that single letter turned a word into a period—in genome parlance, a stop codon. The final 70 words of the sentence were lopped off just as if . . . Yes, just like that.

Mäntyranta didn't make more EPO than you or I. In fact, he had lower than normal quantities circulating in his body. But thanks to the misspelling in his EPOR gene, he was exquisitely sensitive to EPO, churning out fresh red blood cells at the slightest provocation. His rare mutation resulted in his EPOR receptor urging his body to make more red blood cells even when EPO was virtually undetectable. In Mäntyranta's case, his blood lab values were roughly 50 percent higher than a normal man's. Those extra red blood cells likely provided a huge boost in endurance. For comparison, bike racers use EPO to get what's known as their hematocrit up to 50. That means half the volume of your blood is made up of oxygen-toting red cells. Mäntyranta's hematocrit was an astonishing 68—red cells comprised more than two-thirds of his blood.

Some cautions are in order. With rare exceptions, we can't trace athletic talents back to single genes, say one gene for speed, one for strength, another for endurance. The reality is that hundreds or thousands of genes are collaborating in bewilderingly complex patterns to shape each person's athletic potential. Mäntyranta's genetically endowed endurance is one of those exceptions. Even his story is more complicated than a single gene. Higher than normal hematocrits carry big risks for most people, from the unpleasant and inconvenient, such as heat intolerance and joint pain, to the catastrophic including blood clots and strokes. Nevertheless, for at least five generations, some of Mäntyranta's relatives who've inherited the same mutation have lived healthy, long lives with hematocrits that could kill other people. It's likely that a combination of additional genetic variations in that family, along with their lifestyles in rural Finland, somehow protected them. Cranking up a random athlete's hematocrit to a Mäntyrantaian 68 is probably a very bad and dangerous idea.

Most of Eero Mäntyranta's story is well-settled: He had a very rare genetic variation that gave him an off-the-charts level of red cells in his blood, which translated into a massive advantage in sports where endurance is crucial. He was a very successful cross-country skier. What's less clear is what to make of these facts.

Critics of anti-doping cite Mäntyranta's favorable gene as reason to allow artificial enhancements in sport. As one group of authors wrote: "This example reveals the importance of inherited characteristics for performance. Yet, it is treated very differently by conventional sports ethics policies when compared with for example pharmacological aids, even though neither example is 'earned' by the athlete. Apparently, prevailing sports ethics is unconcerned about this contradiction since 'natural' genetic variation is considered to be an acceptable (or irrelevant) inequality, whereas artificial enhancement is not."[3]

Kayser and colleagues miss a step in their reasoning. It would be inconsistent to accept inherited talents while rejecting PEDs *if the only differences that mattered were earned ones.* But, as my imaginary contest with LeBron James showed, "unearned" natural talents can and should make some difference. Are inherited characteristics—"natural" genetic variations—important for performance? Of course. It would be foolish to think otherwise. Inherited characteristics don't explain everything, however. A closer look at Mäntyranta's career suggests that the story is more complicated. If his inherited advantage were so important, we'd expect him to dominate his sport. We'd expect that dominance to be especially obvious in the longer events for which endurance would be most decisive.

But Mäntyranta didn't win all the races he entered. In 1964, his best year by far, he took two golds in the Winter Olympics at Innsbruck, Austria: in the 15- and 30-km cross-country events. He also finished first in the 15-km competition in the Finnish national championship and three other major races that year. But, curiously, he was not nearly as successful in the longest Olympic race, the 50, where he finished an undistinguished ninth though that's where his inherited advantage should have been most decisive.

Before that, in the 1960 Squaw Valley Olympic Games, he finished at the back of the pack in the 15-km competition. By 1968 in Grenoble he won two medals in individual races—a silver and a bronze—but no golds. In the 50-km race he came in 15th. By the 1972 Sapporo Games, the best he could do was 19th place in the 30-km event. He failed to finish the 50-km race. That year he also earned the distinction of becoming the first Finnish athlete to be caught doping—amphetamines, in the national championship. He later acknowledged taking hormones as well—presumably steroids—but said it was prior to their prohibition. (The International Olympic Committee didn't ban steroids until 1967.) On the slim evidence available it's impossible to say how much of his success was due to his unusual genetics, how much to his dedication, and how much to steroids or amphetamines.

The story of Eero Mäntyranta's inherited edge in endurance turns out to be much less straightforward than critics seem to think. Except for one terrific year, 1964, before steroids were banned, he was not dominant in his sport. And then there's the curious puzzle of his relative lack of success in the event for which endurance should matter most of all, the 50-km race. Vesa Tikander, of the Sports Library of Finland, reports "Mäntyranta was always considered a 'sprinter' as far as cross-country skiers go. He won his best results in 15- and 30-km races and was never at ease in the 50-km marathon event." [Personal communication]

Mäntyranta was a gifted and successful elite skier and, by all reports, a good and likable man. His family's genetic propensity to make an excess of red cells likely contributed to his success. But that inherited edge did not allow him to blow away his competitors year after year. It was one of a multitude of inherited factors—natural talents—that shaped his potential. He developed those talents through rigorous training, mastering technique and tactics, and competing with heart and courage.

Critics offer Mäntyranta as evidence that the playing field is never level.[4] Of course they're right about that. We don't all inherit precisely the same athletic abilities. The "biological inequality" they point to is undeniable. The important question, though, is what to make of the ubiquitous inequalities in talents and what the answer means for the ethics of doping. Mäntyranta himself dismissed the significance of his presumed genetic advantage according to David Epstein's account in his book *The Sports Gene*. Mäntyranta insisted that his success was attributable to his determination and will, not his abundance of red blood cells.[5]

EARNED AND UNEARNED

I believe that at the heart of what we care about in sport is the combination of natural talents, the dedication and discipline to perfect those talents, and the courage to test yourself against an external standard, be it your competitor, a measure of distance or height, or the clock. This is true for the full range of people participating in sport, from the Olympic swimmer to the Little Leaguer to the lonely cyclist trying to go as far and as fast as he did last year despite what increasing age does to our physical capacities. (In my case, I try to ride my age in miles, so every year the ride gets longer. I reserve the right to change to kilometers, if necessary.)

The critics I cited above are unhappy that natural talents play such a significant role in sport. They claim that since both doping and natural talents are unearned, they should be treated exactly the same. Either we should permit doping, or we should neutralize somehow the advantages of natural talents. This is the back door to doping. There's also a front door: Some critics claim that athletes should be allowed to use artificial enhancements to level the playing field by bringing their talents up to match those of their competitors.[6]

Anti-doping critics' first assumption begins innocently enough: *Whatever advantage athletes get from either their genes or by doping is unearned.* True. The next step is to claim that *the difference between something that is earned rather than unearned is meaningful and important.* This is often true. We admire a musician who has perfected her violin playing through thousands of hours of practice. But that's not the whole story.

Imagine two buckets labeled "earned" and "unearned." Now take factors that affect performance in sport and decide into which bucket they go. A gene that enhances endurance? Clearly unearned. A course of EPO injections that do the same? Again, unearned. A runner who's improved her time after a grueling training regimen? That seems "earned," but something's not quite right. There's abundant scientific evidence that individuals respond to training in different ways, based on innate factors beyond their control. Perhaps we should think of a person's responsiveness to training as a kind of natural talent. It's certainly no more "earned" than her physiology. At the same time, we have good reason to admire her dedication. If I have to choose, I'm tossing it into the "earned" bucket. But I realize that her success—or lack of it—is affected by her genes all the way through. Two sprinters may run equally fast at the beginning, train equally hard, and end up with very different times in the end.

Cycling demands a variety of abilities: brief bursts of power in sprints; the ability to sustain maximum intensity, sometimes for more than an hour, in time trials; and the endurance to peddle up steep mountain slopes. To race is to suffer. To prepare to race—to train—is also to suffer. Lungs ache, legs burn, your entire body screams "stop!" But the will of great competitors demands they complete whatever task they've taken on despite the pain and exhaustion.

In anyone's book, athletes should receive credit for their dedication and their willingness to endure pain in order to perfect their abilities. Suffering on behalf of a worthy goal is admirable. We should reward dedication and courage. But here it gets complicated. People don't all experience pain in precisely the same way. At identical levels of training, different individuals may make different amounts of the neurotransmitters that signal "this hurts!" They may have a greater or lesser number of receptors—the docks to which the molecular pain signals attach themselves. Some people will experience more pain; some less. The individual's genes affect every step in this process. Has the person who is less sensitive to pain failed to "earn" their success as much as someone who is acutely sensitive to it?

Or perhaps one athlete had parents who taught her to persevere and whose efforts were rewarded with success, so that the dedication required for training became second nature for her, while another would-be athlete's life experiences led her to expect frustration and failure at every turn. Does the second athlete deserve more credit than the first if she persists in the face of disapproval and disappointment?

Sorting out what is genuinely "earned" from what's determined by a person's inherited capacities and life experiences is as much a conceptual as an empirical challenge. We can agree that virtues such as dedication and courage should be encouraged and admired, even if we're far from understanding how much credit to give the individual's willpower and how much to the luck of the genetic and developmental draw.

But are all "unearned" differences—inherited abilities, equipment, drugs—ethically the same for sport? Only if you believe that the talents athletes are born with are indistinguishable from anabolic steroids, EPO, and other performance-enhancing drugs. So let's add a wrinkle to the me-versus-LeBron experiment: Suppose I got hold of an amazing technological boost that enabled me to play as well as LeBron. (I can't imagine what combination of performance enhancing drugs could possibly bridge the chasm between us, but this is an absurd hypothetical after all.) According to anti-doping critics, inherited talents should be regarded the same way we treat artificial enhancements, so whatever miracle drugs I've taken to get up to LeBron's level are perfectly okay. The difference, they imply, should be determined by who has *earned* their performance. Suppose I slightly outwork

LeBron—he took off the occasional Sunday but I never relented. If I outscore him do I deserve my victory? Or is winning with artificial enhancements contrary to the values of sport?

Citing Eero Mäntyranta as an example, critics claim that people no more deserve their success when it's due to their natural talents than they would by doping because neither talents nor doping are "earned." And, they continue, if we tolerate differences in "unearned" natural talents we should be open to allowing athletes to dope. My imaginary match with LeBron James suggests something different: that extraordinary natural talents aren't merely tolerated; they're a fundamental part of what people love about sport.

Let's say the Mäntyranta story was simpler. Imagine what would happen if a single genetic mutation gave whoever had it a completely decisive edge over everyone else in a particular sport. Imagine that Mäntyranta was half again faster than all other cross-country skiers, even if he didn't train nearly as hard as his competitors. In time, I suspect, people would lose interest in competing against him. Perhaps separate competitions would be set up for those with and without inherited polycythemia. Nordic skiing would look more like wrestling and weightlifting with separate competitions for different categories of athletes except the criterion would be hematocrit rather than bodyweight. We want interesting contests, and we want athletes to be able to compete on a playing field that is roughly level except for the natural gifts, honed by dedication, that athletes bring to the competition.

It's true that sport bans "pharmacological aids" but not genetic differences even though neither is earned. But labeling this a "contradiction" assumes there are no relevant differences between winning thanks to an edge provided by drugs and winning because of superior natural talent. Torbjörn Tännsjö, a Swedish philosopher wrote: " . . . in sport we should allow that people level out their inborn differences. We should allow all sorts of (safe) medical and genetic methods of enhancement of athletes. This would pave the way for more exciting competitions and for the possibility that anyone who wants to do so can take part in them on equal terms. And at last we would come to grips with the problem of elitism in sport."[7] (p113) His colleague and frequent co-author, Claudio Tamburrini, tells us where to look: " . . . as genetic modifications probably will level out differences in performance capacity established by birth, athletes' initial conditions will be more equal than they are at present. Thus . . . sport competitions will probably turn out to be fairer . . . there will be more room for morality in this enhanced new (sport) world."[8] (p234)

Tännsjö and Tamburrini would use genetic enhancements to level out differences in natural talents by raising the less talented to the level of their competition. But there's another direction to go: down. We could make it harder for more talented athletes.

DISPENSE WITH TALENT ENTIRELY?

Max Mehlman, a leading expert on health law and public policy, is pessimistic about sport's ability to rein in genetic enhancement and concerned about the intrusiveness of previous efforts to control drugs in sport. Most of the alternatives to testing he sees aren't terribly attractive. He mentions the possibility that sport could simply abandon its ethical ideals, or merely pay them lip service with no serious effort to enforce a ban on genetic enhancement.

But then, Mehlman offers another idea: Sport could "reject talent as an acceptable basis for differences in performance, regardless of how the talent was acquired."[9] (p222) Consider for a moment the merits of his proposal. No matter what was done to enhance an athlete's abilities with genetic manipulation or genetic selection or with drugs, it wouldn't matter a whit. Raw talent, whether it was inherited from someone's parents or amped up with drugs or genetic manipulations, would have nothing to do with success in sport. When doping won't provide any competitive advantage, athletes will lose interest in it. We'd be rewarding athletes who've earned their success through hard work and perseverance. Lack of ability—however acquired—would no longer be an impediment to athletic triumph. (This idea also has the merit of qualifying me as a true expert: I probably know as much about the lack of athletic talent as anyone.)

Most people who love sport value preparation, dedication, discipline, perseverance, the willingness to put in thousands of hours and gallons of sweat in the quest to perfect talent. Mehlman would simply remove unearned talents from the equation. All that would count is what people have to work for. He offers three arguments for his proposal. First, he claims that science's growing abilities to manipulate and select for athletic gifts will overwhelm old-fashioned differences in natural talents. Prediction is always hazardous. Gene therapy—genetic manipulation directed against diseases—is finally coming of age, but it's been slow to arrive, can be very risky, and its results are far from predictable. The era of natural talents is not yet over. I'm much less confident than Mehlman that science will soon, if ever, have the power to sweep away all biological distinctions that matter in sport.

New forms of gene editing such as CRISPR Cas9 offer far more powerful tools for genetic manipulation. But using them to create superathletes faces two obstacles. First, the techniques have a way to go before they are reliable and safe. Those uncertainties and risks, along with other reasons that make us uneasy about tinkering with human embryos or gametes, are slowing the rush to create human superathletes. The second reason is sheer complexity. Tinkering with one or a handful of genes won't give you a great athlete. Except for genes directly linked to particular diseases, the power of a single gene to determine a complex human trait is usually diffuse and indirect. There may be rare exceptions—remember Eero Mäntyranta—but successful athletes are never made by a single gene. Still, gene editing deserves to be closely watched for its possible impact on sport.

Genetic testing for sports talent has little more to offer. The big story so far has been the test for variants in the ACTN3 gene that appear to be correlated with the proportion of fast-twitch to slow-twitch muscle fibers. More fast-twitch fibers may mean quicker, more powerful contractions; more slow-twitch fibers may translate into increased endurance. In its early days, you could have a sample of DNA tested for $129. When the company that first marketed the test said it would test only adults, not children, I doubted this policy would survive. For one thing, all that the lab saw were cells from a cheek swab stuck into a test tube. It had no way of knowing whether the cells came from you, your child—or some kid whose budding career you hope to promote and make a fortune off of. The company was probably testing children even when their policy prohibited it. For another, the market for testing children and adolescents is much larger than for adults. The early years are crucial for promising athletes. When parents, coaches, or teams are deciding which young athletes to invest their time and resources in, they'd like to know sooner rather than later who is the best bet. A test that could predict which of the more than two million kids playing Little League have the genes to become a major leaguer would attract lots of customers.

But, so far, there's no evidence that the ACTN3 test, or any other genetic test, can pick out the most athletically talented.[10]

At least, not any better than watching the young person play. The best piece of technology for identifying a talented young sprinter is still a stopwatch. You can pick up a nifty one on Amazon for around forty dollars and use it over and over—a much better deal than $99 a pop (the current price) for a test unlikely to tell you much about your child's athletic future.

Mehlman argues that we have neither the legal and policy tools, nor the will to create and deploy them, to deter people from engaging in genetic manipulation and selection. On this point he's mostly correct. Some of the ways people might seek genetic enhancement may strike most of us as really bad ideas—parents trying to create superathletes through pre-implantation genetic selection and manipulation, for example.[11] But bad, even terrible ideas are not always illegal. And America's reluctance to regulate parents' choices (other than the decision whether to have an abortion) and the practices of the infertility industry leave a broad and wild territory on the frontiers of reproduction.[12]

One other point: Mehlman assumes that efforts to detect genetic manipulation are doomed to be intolerably intrusive and ultimately futile. He may be giving too little credit to the ingenuity of the researchers developing methods to uncover genetic tinkering. Until recently, scientists had nowhere to turn for support for such research. With the modest funds now available, some strides are being made to identify stigmata left by genetic manipulation. The outcome of this particular contest is far from certain, but the home team is now in the game.

Finally, Mehlman offers the familiar distinction between earned and unearned determinants of success on the playing field and argues that only earned ones should be allowed to count: "Neither natural talent nor good fortune are earned or deserved."[9 (p213)] He has two big problems here. We've talked about the first: deciding what counts as truly "earned." The second is even more daunting: coming up with a practical scheme for neutralizing the impact of differences in natural talents.

THE HARRISON BERGERON OLYMPICS?

Mehlman offers a brief sketch of how this could be done: "Athletes would be tested before competing and handicapped according to their native ability. This would not be performance testing, because that would conflate talent with effort, thereby handicapping athletes who worked hard at the same level as those with inherited or installed ability. Instead, some method would have to be found to measure pure ability—most likely a sophisticated combination of phenotypic and genetic markers."[9] [(p222)]

By "installed" ability Mehlman means genetic manipulation. "Gene doping" as it's called has received attention far out of proportion to its likely impact on sport in the near future. The genetic markers he refers to presumably would be for genes associated with athletic talents, like the ACTN3 gene. Your "phenotype" on the other hand is everything that can be observed: Are you tall or short, thickly muscled or scrawny, graceful or a complete klutz? But we don't know much about which genes to tinker with or test for, so any installing or testing likely won't have a significant impact on sport for a long time.

So, how do we assess natural talents, and how do we handicap gifted competitors? Some assessments will be easier than others. Tall people have an advantage in sports such as basketball and volleyball. No one "earns" her or his height. It's determined by a combination of genes and environment—like being well-fed and avoiding serious diseases. If anyone deserves credit, it would be your parents. According to Mehlman, height should not be permitted to affect one's success in sport. The assessment is

straightforward: simply measure everyone. But, how do you neutralize the impact of height in a sport such as basketball? And
not all natural advantages will be as unambiguous and easy to
measure as height.

Measuring the relative proportions of fast-twitch and slow-
twitch muscle fibers might help us assess who has natural advantages for sports that require strength and explosive bursts of
power versus those for which endurance is more important. But
just how "natural" can these proportions be when there is evidence that training can alter them?[13] Untangling "unearned"
natural talents from the effects of perseverance and smart training will be the quandary that keeps on giving.

And then there are talents that defy our best efforts to dis-
tinguish between what's earned and unearned. Take baseball.
The gracefulness of a shortstop darting to his right, backhanding
the ball despite a bad hop, leaping and turning to make a strong,
accurate throw to first base to get the runner. A third baseman
with the courage to stand close to the batter and the reflexes to
get his glove on a wicked liner. A savvy catcher who studies hitters' tendencies, uncovers their vulnerabilities, and calls for just
the right pitch in the right location.

That shortstop's grace, arm strength, and accuracy are not
purely natural gifts; they've been perfected through years of
practice and training. The third baseman's reflexes may be mostly
determined by his genes, but where does his courage come from?
The catcher's dedication may be earned, but what about his superior intellect? If we believe that intelligence is an advantage in
some sport, must we test for it as well so that we can handicap
the smarter players because they haven't "earned" their intellect?
That seems to be the direction Mehlman's proposal leads.

Kurt Vonnegut's short story "Harrison Bergeron," in his collection *Welcome to the Monkey House*, imagines a country where

no one is permitted to be more talented than anyone else. Diana Moon Glampers, the Handicapper General, has her minions hang weights on the legs of talented dancers and fix noise-emitting devices on the heads of smart people so that they can't think without interruption.[14] Should our shortstop be obliged to wear weights around his ankles, the third baseman weights on his wrists, and the catcher one of those thought-interrupters? Leveling the playing field by handicapping people with superior natural talents is a strategy with limited appeal. Non-elite golfers have handicaps so that people of different abilities can have interesting competitions. But professional golfers compete without them.

Imagine a case in which an overweight person wants to run the 100-meter sprint. The aspiring sprinter provides medical testimony that his excess weight is caused by a glandular abnormality, so he doesn't "deserve" to be fat. He protests that the sleek, lithe athletes running against him have the unearned advantage of carrying many fewer pounds to the finish line. So, he suggests, shouldn't they be laden with weights to neutralize their natural advantage over him? If Mehlman's reasoning prevails, every race, every sports contest, would have to be handicapped to the level of the least talented participant.

The idea that we should impose handicaps to eradicate the advantages of natural talents in sport is an easy target. But working through the implications of the proposal helps illuminate why it goes wrong. The fault lies in its assumption that unearned, natural talents are somehow unfair and must always be redressed. I'm curious to see how this same principle would work if it was applied to the institutions in which the critics work. The universities and law and medical schools I know try to select students and faculty who are smart and dedicated. In those hallowed halls one does not often hear arguments that it's unfair to exclude the dull and uncurious just because they are that way naturally.

John Rawls, the esteemed political philosopher who developed the theory of justice as fairness, explicitly rejected the notion that justice requires redress for all inequalities. Rawls was acutely aware that people differ in the talents they bring to the world. But he was an advocate for justice, not for leveling.

Rawls wrote: "[A]fter a game one often says that the losing side deserved to win. Here one does not mean that the victors are not entitled to claim the championship, or whatever spoils go to the winner. One means instead that the losing team displayed to a higher degree the skills and qualities that the game calls forth, and the exercise of which gives the sport its appeal. Therefore the losers truly deserved to win but lost out as a result of bad luck, or from other contingencies that caused the contest to miscarry."[15] (p314) The distinction here that the critics miss is between *entitlement* and *moral worth*. The winners of the contest, as long as they didn't cheat, are entitled to their victory and whatever rewards come with it. The losers may have played better, and deserve to be admired for the worthiness of the performance. But they still lost. As I've said before: Sport is not a morality contest where only the virtuous win.

MARVEL AND ADMIRE

Knowing who *deserves* to win requires that we have a clear idea about what *ought* to count and, therefore, what's fair and unfair. If the judges for Olympic figure skating awarded the gold medal according to which contestant had the most revealing costume— or the most sequins or feathers—that's obviously unfair. Or suppose they were bribed, or favored certain countries' skaters, or flipped a coin. Everyone knows this would be wrong. The International Skating Union's Rule 353 takes five pages to describe the criteria judges are supposed to use in scoring skaters' performances.[16] The details are head-achingly complicated, but the two constants are how challenging a skater's program is and how skillfully it was executed. That's what figure skating values. That's what should determine who wins.

Those are the two dimensions along which we measure all great sportspersons. We marvel and wonder at their extraordinary talents. And we admire the qualities through which those talents were honed and perfected. Marvel and wonder. Admire. Both dimensions are there in every sports performance.

If you're inclined toward cynicism—if you're paying attention at all—sport provides abundant reasons for regarding it as exemplifying much of the worst in human nature. Athletes can be preening, coddled, and vain with a reservoir of moral integrity shallow enough to be drained in one gulp. Owners of professional teams can be narcissistic and greedy. Some college coaches rip through programs leaving a trail of suppurating wounds in their wake. Gamblers—legal and illegal—wage staggering sums on sporting events; sometimes they find athletes willing to take bribes to fix games.

Come to think of it, just about every human institution worth our time and attention has the same problem of providing a platform from which the morally bankrupt can break the hearts of the upstanding. Think business and politics; also marriage, friendship, and families. Marriage may be the triumph of hope over experience that skeptics claim, but plenty of people try it, some regret it later, but others make it work and are glad they succeeded—most of the time at least. When my father was asked if he'd ever considered divorce he'd reply, "Divorce? No. Murder? That's another story."

These institutions and practices arise to meet vital human aspirations and needs. Whatever their flaws, and however often we are disappointed when they fail us—or we fail to live up to our own expectations—they would not exist without some plausible belief that our lives, on the whole, are better because of them. Sport, in its failures and its glories, is no different.

NOTES

1. Bradley B. *Values of the Game*. New York: Broadway; 2000. p. 96.
2. de la Chapelle A, Träskelin AL, Juvonen E. Truncated erythropoietin receptor causes dominantly inherited benign human erythrocytosis. *Proc Natl Acad Sci U S A*. 1993 May;90(10):4495–4499.
3. Kayser B, Mauron A, Miah A. Current anti-doping policy: A critical appraisal. *BMC Med Ethics*. 2007;8:1–10.
4. Savulescu J, Foddy B, Clayton M. Why we should allow performance enhancing drugs in sport. *Br J Sports Med*. 2004 Dec;38(6):666–674.
5. Epstein D. *The Sports Gene: Inside the Science of Extraordinary Athletic Performance*. New York: Current; 2014. p. 368.
6. Miah A. Enhanced Athletes? It's Only Natural [Internet]. *Washington Post*. 2008 Aug 3 [cited 2016 Dec 28]. Available from: http://www.washingtonpost.com/wp-dyn/content/article/2008/08/01/AR2008080103060.html.
7. Tännsjö T. Hypoxic air machines: Commentary. *J Med Ethics*. 2005 Feb 1; 31(2):113.
8. Tamburrini CM. What's wrong with genetic inequality? The impact of genetic technology on elite sports and society. *Sport Ethics Philos*. 2007;1(2):229–238.
9. Mehlman M. Genetic enhancement in sport: Ethical, legal and policy concerns. In: Murray TH, Maschke KJ, Wasunna AA, editors. *Performance-Enhancing Technologies in Sports: Ethical, Conceptual, and Scientific Issues*. Baltimore: Johns Hopkins University Press; 2009. p. 205–224.
10. Brooks MA. Genetic testing and youth sports. *JAMA J Am Med Assoc*. 2011;305(10):1033–1034.
11. Sandel MJ. *The Case against Perfection: Ethics in the Age of Genetic Engineering*. Cambridge, MA: Belknap Press; 2007.
12. Murray TH. Stirring the simmering "designer baby" pot. *Science*. 2014 Mar 14;343(6176):1208–1210.

13. Wilson JM, Loenneke JP, Jo E, Wilson GJ, Zourdos MC, Kim J-S. The effects of endurance, strength, and power training on muscle fiber type shifting. *J Strength Cond Res*. 2012 Jun;26(6):1724–1729.
14. Vonnegut K. *Welcome to the Monkey House*. Reprint edition. New York: Paw Prints; 2008.
15. Rawls J. *A Theory of Justice*. Revised edition. Cambridge, MA: Belknap Press; 1999. 560 p.
16. International Skating Union. International Skating Union Special Regulations & Technical Rules Single & Pair Skating [Internet]. 2014 [cited 2016 Aug 8]. Available from: http://static.isu.org/media/166717/2014-special-regulation-sandp-and-ice-dance-and-technical-rules-sandp-and-id_14-09-16.pdf.

Chapter 3

Rules and Meanings

The physical layout of the game is perfectly adjusted to the human skills it is meant to display and call into graceful exercise.

John Rawls on baseball

Golf is perverse. Such a simple game: Knock a ball around until it falls into the correct hole. Yet it drives people nuts. Turns out that hitting the ball straight isn't so easy. A little sidespin, and it may carom off a tree, plunk into water, or come to rest in tall grass or sand.

Happily, there's a remedy.

Unhappily, the tyrants controlling golf tournaments won't let you use it.

Polara Golf designs balls that reduce the consequence for striking one poorly by up to 75 percent. So instead of ping-ponging your ball off trees, you likely will be hitting from the pleasant manicured grass of the fairway. Why does the U.S. Golf Association ban all such balls from tournament play?

The Polara Ultimate Straight ball is a clever piece of technology. Deep dimples along the axis of flight and shallow dimples around the equator make for a ball that flies lower and straighter. Just point the inscribed arrow down the fairway and swing. We're a people who love technology. If it makes it easier, faster or more efficient, terrific. Why, then, does the sport of golf spurn innovative balls that help golfers stay out of the rough and sand traps?

Perhaps it's not a puzzle at all. The ability to hit a ball squarely so that it flies true rather than hooking or slicing is a crucial skill in golf. Doing that consistently is the road to excellence in the sport. The authorities governing golf decided that a ball that flies straight no matter what makes it *too* easy. They reached the same conclusion about clubfaces with deep rectangular grooves that enhance golfers' ability to hit controlled shots out of the tall grass typically growing in the "rough" surrounding the trimmed fairway. Hitting out of the rough is harder; rejecting the clever new clubs can only mean that golf believes it's *supposed to be* harder.

Golf isn't alone. Swimming and speed skating also banned innovative technologies that enabled enhanced performances. Pole-vaulting, on the other hand, welcomed poles made of new materials that allowed athletes to leap ever higher. It's not only new technologies, either. Baseball made it harder for pitchers by lowering the mound. Basketball tinkers regularly with its rules in response to new kinds of athletes and new strategies.

If sport isn't full-on perverse in its ambivalence toward performance-enhancing technologies, it's certainly unusual. Can you imagine a manufacturer turning down a new machine because it cranks out more widgets per hour and makes them more precisely? Or an accounting firm insisting that its employees only use hand-cranked calculators—or an abacus—for all their computations? (Artisan beer and cheesemakers that use old-fashioned methods are increasingly popular, but I don't see the attraction of an artisanal accounting firm.)

A game without rules isn't much of a game at all. Except perhaps for Calvinball, which has just one rule: that you can't use the same rule twice. The late Lee Atwater, a notoriously hard-nosed political operative, noted the similarity between politics and knife fighting. His opponents, he explained, had forgotten the first rule of knife fights: there are no rules.

Still, it's hard to imagine a meaningful contest without rules, even a pie-baking competition. It wouldn't be fair to give one baker a well-regulated modern oven and force the other contestants to use antique broken-down unreliable ones—unless the contest was meant to measure oven technology instead of baking skills.

The central question is whether the rules of a sport are essentially arbitrary, as some commentators claim, or whether they instead reflect some deeper understanding of what the sport means and what it values. If a sport is just what its rules say it is, no more and no less, then it's up to the rulemakers' whims whether to welcome or to ban golf balls and clubs, hinged skates, or buoyant swimsuits. On the other hand, if a sport's rules express widely shared ideas about what's valued in that sport, then decisions about technologies that improve performance must be tested against those values and meanings. We should expect those same values to guide sport's attitudes and rules on anabolic steroids, stimulants, EPO, growth hormone, or any other performance-enhancing drug.[1] Consider how several sports have dealt with change and innovation.

KLAPSKATES AND FAIRNESS AS EQUAL ACCESS

In 1997, Dutch speed skaters began using a skate hinged near the toe that offered distinct biomechanical advantages. Skaters try to keep the full length of their blade in contact with the ice to generate as much force as possible and to avoid dragging their toe. Traditional speed skates required athletes to keep a roughly ninety-degree angle between leg and foot. Klapskates, as they came to be known, allowed skaters to more fully extend their legs, flex their ankles, and push with their feet as if they were running.

The klapskates ignited an international controversy. Skaters wearing them were suddenly whipping Olympians from other countries. Speed skating is as important to the Netherlands as baseball is to America; when skaters from other nations tried to buy klapskates, they complained that the Dutch companies were holding back the "good stuff" and sending them inferior ones. Athletes accustomed to traditional speedskates also had to learn a new technique to take full advantage of the klapskates. Athletes and officials in other countries protested that the skates violated the purity of the sport.[2]

The opposition to klapstakes was based on two distinct claims. The first complaint was unfairness: Dutch athletes had a monopoly on equipment that gave whoever learned to use it well an enormous edge. This was true. Skaters from other nations were unhappy losing to Dutch skaters they were sure were inferior athletes. Technology was trumping talent and dedication. The solution to this unfairness was to allow all speedskaters access to top-of-the-line klapskates. The Dutch skaters' technological advantage soon evaporated.

The second complaint was more subtle and interesting. American sprinter Christine Witty complained that what had been a pure sport was being wrecked by "this machine." Klapskates required modifying one's technique. Some athletes complained that they were easier to use, that skaters unable or unwilling to master traditional speedskates were zipping by them in klapskates. Discipline and technique were devalued; the nature of the sport was being altered. Then again, Witty used the skates in setting a new world record in the 1,000-meter event.

The International Skating Union faced a tough decision. If klapskates were like jetpacks, if the technology overshadowed the talents and discipline at the heart of speed skating, then the ISU should have banned them. If, on the other hand, success on klapskates depended on the same characteristics that mattered for traditional skates—power, endurance, balance, grace, finely honed technique (even if the technique's details were slightly different)—then the ISU had a plausible reason to accept klapskates as a legitimate technical innovation. And that's what it did, though to what extent its decision reflected careful philosophical reflection or the power of the Dutch lobby, we don't know for certain. The skates were legal by the 1998 Nagano Winter Olympics. Motivation matters morally, but messy deliberations sometimes lead to defensible results. My favorite sidelight to the klapskate story is the effort of the ISU president to change the name of the skate because its first syllable rhymes with slang for a sexually transmitted disease.[2] [p195] Hinged skate blades were latecomers, though, compared to the innovations in pole vaulting.

IT'S NOT THE POLE; IT'S THE VAULTER

A.C. Gilbert, the 1908 Olympic pole vault co-champion, described his first pole: a length of cedar taken from a fence and shaped by hand with a drawshave. Gilbert was not happy sharing the gold medal with Edwin Tiffin Cooke, Jr., who had cleared 12 feet 2 inches in a qualifying round. Gilbert reached that same height in the final round, when the best Cooke could do was 11 feet 9 inches. A few months before, Gilbert had set a world record at the US Olympic trials clearing 12 feet ¾ inches using a bamboo pole and planting it in a hole he'd dug that prevented the pole from slipping on the turf. Having your pole skid along the ground had been a common hazard for vaulters.

At the 1908 London Olympics, Gilbert carried a hatchet onto the track and began hacking away at the ground. The English judges would have none of it. They may have been annoyed that the US flag bearer in the Olympic parade had refused to dip his banner to the royal box. Whatever their reasons, they prohibited Gilbert and his fellow vaulters from using this early version of what came to be known as a "plant box." Irritated English officials proved to be no more than a brief hiccup in the history of pole vaulting. With lighter, more flexible bamboo poles replacing heavier unyielding wooden ones, and with holes offering more secure plants, the pole vault was on the verge of a revolution.

Pole-vaulting has long been influenced by changes in equipment and technique. Before 1889, many American competitors could have been more aptly described as pole climbers. They would run with their heavy wooden poles, stick them in the ground in front of the crossbar, then scramble hand over hand up the pole until they reached the bar. That year a rule was instituted forbidding competitors from raising their uppermost hand once the vault was begun, or from bringing the lower hand anywhere above the upper one—in other words, no more climbing. Pole climbing was an early "enhancement" the sport of vaulting firmly rejected.

By the turn of the century, vaulters such as Gilbert began digging holes they could insert their poles into more securely. Before the advent of the hole, which later became a full-fledged box with wooden plant board, bottom and sides, vaulters would drive spikes into the end of the pole to give it better odds of sticking where they put it. The London Olympic judges may have balked in 1908, but by 1924 the modern plant box had taken shape and been incorporated into the rules for the sport.

In what historians of the pole vault regard as its transformational era, the world record was shattered eight times by six different athletes over a span of seven years.[3] This was not the 1960s, when the fiberglass pole came into regular use; rather, the transformation took place from 1904 to 1911, when sturdy, light bamboo poles revolutionized the vault. With less weight to carry down the track, athletes ran faster and with better balance. The fundamental limiting factors in the pole vault are the energy generated by the run-up to the crossbar combined with the height of the grip. A flexible pole allows the vaulter to store energy in the pole by continuing to run as it bends.

Aluminum poles came into vogue around World War II, when bamboo was scarce in the United States. Track and field's international ruling body, the IAAF, had changed its rules in 1936 to permit materials other than wood and bamboo. Aluminum was light but not terribly flexible. Tapered steel and fiberglass poles were available by 1948, but the early fiberglass poles vaulters experimented with in the 1950s had some disconcerting quirks. A pole introduced by a California maker of fiberglass masts for sailboats was said to grow increasingly flexible with use—until it snapped. The 1960 Rome Olympic Games were the last in which any medal was won by a vaulter using old-style metal poles. Not one US Olympic team vaulter used a fiberglass pole that year. But it did not take long for fiberglass and carbon fiber poles to become dominant. In 1963 a single vaulter, John Pennel, broke the world record four times within two months, including the first vault of 17 feet.[4]

From Rome in 1960 to Bob Seagren's vault of 17 feet 8 ½ inches eight years later in Mexico City, the Olympic record increased nearly 15 percent, matching almost exactly the improvement over the forty years prior to 1960. New poles once again revolutionized the sport. Athletes were leaping higher and higher. But the champions were still those individuals with the combination of speed, strength, and grace that had been the winning formula in vaulting since pole climbing was outlawed. R.A. Ganslen offered this caution in his classic book *Mechanics of the Pole Vault*: "The slow or gradual extension of the fiberglass poles is misleading to laymen and creates a catapulting impression. However, the principal advantage of the pole was and is to permit a take-off at maximum speed with a high hand grip and small angle between the pole and the ground . . . an impossibility with a stiff pole."[4 (p41)] He had this to say about success in the event: "Many modern pole vaulters display incredible strength and the speed of sprinters. In the final analysis, speed, strength, and tallness are distinct advantages to the vaulter."[4 (p145)]

SUPER-SLIPPERY SWIMSUITS

Swimming was forced to reexamine what it valued when records began to fall at an unprecedented pace. The 2009 world championships in Rome saw forty-three world record swims. Records were smashed by men and by women in sprints as well as long-distance events. A pair of scientists at Northwestern University considered a variety of explanations: Had the rules changed? Were training methods that much better? Was it because of one or two exceptional swimmers? They compared swimmers to runners, whose times had also improved over the previous twenty years—but nowhere near as dramatically. For example, at the end of those two decades, men's times running the 400-meter dash were 2.85 percent faster; in the 100-meter freestyle swimmers improved by 5.86 percent—more than twice as much. Whether they compared men or women, long or short distances, swimmers' speeds increased far more than runners'.[5]

The only changes that could account for the difference were the suits. Manufacturers were producing revolutionary racing swimsuits made of polyurethane that covered nearly the whole body. The material was impermeable to water. Because the suits fit so snugly, they trapped pockets of air making the swimmer more buoyant. More buoyancy means less muscle and bone to drag through the water. (Water offers roughly 780 times the resistance of air.) The suits also smoothed and shaped the body, reducing drag. And they were hydrophobic—they repelled water—allowing the wearer to slip through the water.[6]

The suits had drawbacks. It could take half an hour to put one on; they cost about $500 each; and they lasted for just a few races. And you might not get access to the best ones: Different manufacturers competed to make the fastest suits—and provide them exclusively to the athletes they sponsored. So if your sponsor was behind the curve, your odds of winning plummeted. But the sport of swimming had concerns about these suits beyond equal access. An official of FINA, the international governing body for swimming, defended the proposed rules changes banning the impermeable, full-body suits: "Swimming has traditionally been a sport where equipment has been secondary to individual talent and determination. With the swimsuits introduced in 2008, equipment became primary, enabling athletes of lesser ability to compete on equal terms with the best-conditioned, hardest-working athletes in the sport. That is why the mandate for change was clear."[7]

This is what really bothered people, swimmers as well as officials: The new suits threatened to change the meaning of the sport. Swimming was now rewarding muscled, stocky athletes who paddled on top of the water rather than sleek bodies slicing through it. The new swimsuits threatened to alter what swimming valued. The point of the new rules that banned many swimsuits was to restore and preserve the values and meaning of the sport.

The values at stake here don't belong exclusively to swimming. Other sports object to equipment that allows "athletes of lesser ability" to be successful against "the best-conditioned, hardest-working athletes in the sport." This is further evidence that sports value athletes' natural talents along with the dedication that allows athletes to perfect their technique and skills.

The rules of each sport reward particular combinations of natural talents, perfected through dedication and hard work.[8] Sports pursue that goal by establishing what sorts of differences are permitted to determine the outcome and, at least as important, what differences ought *not* be permitted to affect an athlete's results. Swimming declared that body-shaping, buoyant, slippery swimsuits should not allow athletes of lesser talent to swim faster than competitors with superior gifts and work ethics. Swimming and other sports likewise believe that performance-enhancing drugs should not be allowed to influence who wins and who loses, lest athletes with inferior talent and discipline— but more potent drugs—triumph over their more talented and dedicated competitors.

BASKETBALL: AS THE PLAYERS CHANGE, SO MUST THE RULES

Changes in the rules of sport, when they are wise, keep alive what the sport is meant to value under the onslaught of changes in equipment, tactics, and, sometimes, the athletes themselves. By 1945, as basketball players grew taller and more athletic, a rule was created to ban a newly invented practice: goaltending, in which a tall player stands under the basket and swats away an opponent's shot just before it can go through the hoop. Very tall players also could dominate on offense, so an area under the basket was defined and offensive players were forbidden to remain in it for more than three consecutive seconds. By 1967, college basketball tried to ban the dunk, a rule that the famously candid coach Al McGuire attributed to fear of UCLA's dominant center, Lew Alcindor, later known as Kareem Abdul-Jabbar.

By 1961, the short-lived American Basketball League introduced the three-point shot into professional basketball. Shots made from beyond an arc painted a good distance from the basket were awarded three points rather than two. Later, the American Basketball Association adopted a similar rule. Only in the 1979–1980 season did the NBA incorporate the three-pointer. The shot was used rarely in its early years until players developed their skill with it and coaches began to see its strategic possibilities. In his first five NBA seasons, Michael Jordon never attempted as many as a hundred three-pointers—and made fewer than 20 percent. In his sixth season, 1989–1990, Jordon tossed up 245, making almost 38 percent of them. The shot became an important part of his repertoire for the remainder of his career.

George Mikan, legendary big man and co-founder of the ABA, championed the three-pointer. He is said to have justified it as a way to open up the court, give smaller players more opportunities to score, and make the game more exciting for fans. Mikan understood how large muscular players could dominate; his strength, determination, and lethal hook shot with either hand prompted the league to double the width of the lane from six to twelve feet, which came to be known as the "Mikan rule." Mikan also bore some responsibility for the shot clock, which requires teams to attempt a shot that at least hits the rim within 24 seconds of taking possession of the ball. The Fort Wayne Pistons beat Mikan's Minneapolis Lakers, 19–18, on 22 November 1950. The teams made eight baskets between them. The Pistons calculated—correctly—that their best chance was to slow the game to a crawl. But it made for a boring, inartistic contest. The league instituted a shot clock in 1954.

George Mikan and Kareem Abdul-Jabbar are just two examples of how basketball has had to change its rules to keep the sport interesting. When players or strategies change, the game must adjust. Jack Ramsey, the legendary basketball coach, likened his sport to ballet: "a graceful sweep and flow of patterned movement, counterpointed by daring and imaginative flights of solitary brilliance. It is a dance which begins with opposition contesting every move. But in the exhilaration of a great performance, the opposition vanishes. The dancer does as he pleases. The game is unified action up and down the floor."9 (p108–109)

Steph Curry is likely the most balletic player of his era and may be the greatest three-point shooter of all time. Thanks to his extraordinary combination of accuracy, quickness, and grace, Curry's team, the Golden State Warriors, won the 2015 NBA championship. Curry is a joy to watch—unless you're rooting for the other team, as I was, or are repelled by his habit of chewing on his dangling mouth guard. As the Warriors and other teams rely increasingly on the three-point shot, their opponents are closely guarding the best shooters out past the three-point line. So basketball yet again adapts to new kinds of players and new strategies of play, refining its rules as it goes. The Cleveland Cavaliers, who lost to Curry's team in 2015, figured out how to beat Golden State for the NBA championship in 2016, becoming the first team in NBA history to come back from a three-games-to-one deficit in the finals.

ARE THE RULES OF SPORT ARBITRARY?
IS THAT A PROBLEM?

If there is a more arbitrary number in sport than baseball's stipulated distance from the pitcher's rubber to home plate of 60 feet, 6 inches, I can't think of it. Why not round it off to 60 feet for heaven's sake? Or stretch it out to 61 feet?

To be sure, there is a story about how this odd number came to be. The often-repeated claim that it was supposed to be 66 feet but someone misread the plan is likely false. That, however, leaves the stranger conclusion that this bizarre number was chosen intentionally.

Curiously, it works. Neither pitcher nor batter has an overwhelming advantage at this distance. A 90-mile-per-hour-plus fastball reaches home plate four-tenths of a second after it leaves the pitcher's hand. The batter must determine what speed it's traveling, whether it will curve or drop, if it will be a strike, and—if the decision is to swing—accelerate the bat toward the ball. Good hitters take from 14 hundredths to 18 hundredths of a second to swing, leaving them a quarter of a second to decide what to do. Contact hitters are typically quicker than power hitters, so they have a few thousandths of a second longer to decide whether and where to swing.

Move the mound and rubber 20 feet closer to the plate, and hitters' decision time would be sliced from a quarter of a second to a tenth of a second. No contest. Move them 20 feet farther away, and pitchers might as well be throwing batting practice.

The renowned philosopher and lover of baseball John Rawls wrote a letter giving reasons why baseball is the best of all games: "First: the rules of the game are in equilibrium: that is, from the start, the diamond was made just the right size, the pitcher's mound just the right distance from home plate, etc., and this makes possible the marvelous plays, such as the double play. The physical layout of the game is perfectly adjusted to the human skills it is meant to display and call into graceful exercise."[10]

The rules of a sport such as baseball do more than merely put all players on a level footing. As Rawls recognized, they create a balance, a tension, among competitors that permits the combination of skills particular to that sport to be exhibited, to mark the difference between success and failure, victory and defeat.

If this is true, there must be some collective wisdom residing in those who understand the sport that constrains the rulemakers. Suppose the people in charge of baseball decided to move the pitcher's mound half the distance to home plate. With pitches being released 30 feet away, hitters would have no time to swing a bat; they would be reduced to bunting—if they could get their bat on the ball at all. Baseball would be reduced to a pitcher, a catcher, seven infielders, and a hapless batter. Everyone who loves or plays baseball would be outraged. The folks who imposed this stupid rule would be run out of the game in disgrace.

The rules of baseball, like the rules of other sports, have been modified over time. But it's a mistake to assume that those alterations were arbitrary in any ethically troublesome sense. The height of the pitcher's rubber was lowered from 15 to 10 inches when giants such as Bob Gibson routinely intimidated and overwhelmed batters. In 1968 Gibson's earned-run average was an astonishing 1.12 per game, with 13 complete-game shutouts in 34 starts. That same year Don Drysdale pitched 58 ⅔ consecutive scoreless innings. By 1969, the rubber was five inches lower, reducing the pitcher's advantage.

Writers who criticize the rules of sport for being arbitrary are confused about the concept. Yes, there are occasions when arbitrariness is morally offensive, even wicked. Rewarding one person while pummeling another for no reason other than you feel like it is arbitrary, wrong, and completely without justification. Setting the distance between the pitcher's rubber and home plate at 60 feet 6 inches is also arbitrary. But perfectly reasonable if your goal is to sustain a competitive balance between pitcher and hitter.

Imagine if we took to heart the criticism that this distance was arbitrary, and we decided to leave it up to the pitchers where they would stand. I've put this question to a pitcher. He volunteered that he'd move right up to the catcher. Effective—and boring.

An "arbitrary" rule in sport has to satisfy two conditions. First, it must be as reasonable as any other standard that might have been chosen—60 feet 6 inches is not notably worse a distance than any other. Second, the rule should help to preserve what's meaningful and valued in that sport. Whether it's the height of the pitcher's mound, the three-second lane, the ban on goaltending, or the three-point arc, the rules of each sport are justified by their success at protecting meaning and value—including the life and health of those who play the sport.

The standard goal in soccer is eight feet tall and 24 feet wide. I suggested (facetiously) to some European critics of anti-doping that they make the goal 48 feet wide; Americans, I said, would find the game more exciting if more goals were scored. The thought horrified them. Widening the goal would make scoring too easy. Goalies would have to leave a huge section of the goal completely unguarded. The goalie's skill and savvy would be neutralized. Strikers could just aim for the vast openings no goalie could possibly cover. A hockey-size goal, on the other hand, at four-by-six feet, would make it nearly impossible to score. Very young soccer players start out with a much smaller target, 4.5-by-9 feet, for the same reason. The goalies are smaller, less agile, and cover less ground. A full-size goal would be too much area to patrol effectively. The nets in soccer and ice hockey are the size they are because they create a tension, a real contest between goalie and shooter, just as 60 feet 6 inches allows pitchers and hitters to test their skills against one another.[11]

The rules of a sport tell us what that sport values. Sometimes, it's the safety of participants and spectators. The javelin, really a sort of spear, was redesigned to make it more nose-heavy so it wouldn't fly as far and would stick in the ground rather than skid along it. The record with the old javelin was 104.8 meters—nearly 344 feet, almost the length of a football field including end zones. The change made the distance thrown easier to measure. It also eased concerns about spearing people at the other end of the stadium.

Rules in sport promote other values as well. They may try to assure that a competition is interesting by matching roughly equally capable athletes or teams against one another, and a sport may have rules for ending a game early when one team has dominated. Rules in sport have an essential function: to select from among the myriad differences among players the ones that should affect outcomes. Raw physical attributes are one source of differences. Because basketball is a game played largely in the air, height is a crucial advantage. All other things equal, taller players have an edge. In football, it helps to be a behemoth to play on the offensive or defensive line. That same body would be an enormous disadvantage for competing in the marathon or playing shortstop, where speed and endurance and quickness and agility are prized qualities. In addition to body type, people vary hugely in their skills—vision, reaction time, mobility, gracefulness and so on. Athletes also differ in how well they master strategies, which is how some aging athletes manage to perform better than their younger, more physically gifted competitors.

The relationship between rules and values in sport goes both ways. In a healthy sport, what we value gets written into and reinforced in the rules. And if you want to know what a sport values, look carefully at its rules. It turns out that a healthy sport's "arbitrary" rules aren't arbitrary at all. They are inextricably tethered to its values and meanings.

The combinations of body type, raw abilities, skills, and strategic savvy that influence success can differ greatly from sport to sport. For all that variety, though, every sport values certain traits of character—call them virtues—such as perseverance, courage, dedication, hard work, and the willingness to endure discomfort in the pursuit of excellence. This is one reason so many people who play and love sport are uncomfortable with the use of performance-enhancing drugs. Whatever it is that we admire about athletic excellence, the size of one's medicine cabinet doesn't fit into the picture.

RULES, MEANINGS AND TECHNOLOGIES

The question, of course, is whether drugs, genetic manipulation, or other enhancement technologies ought to be prohibited. Some critics of doping control argue that sports' rules should accommodate or even encourage biomedical enhancements. Performance-enhancing drugs, they say, are just one of the many technologies athletes use to improve their performance, and it's unfair and irrational to ban them arbitrarily.

Of course, sports ban technologies all the time, such as golf balls that fly too straight and body-clinging, impermeable, water-repelling swimsuits. They also welcome (eventually) some new technologies, such as bamboo and then fiberglass vaulting poles. Drawing lines in a chaotic world isn't easy. You should be able to offer good reasons why some sort of line must be drawn in the first place, and why drawing it here rather than there is a reasonable choice.

"NATURAL" IS IMPORTANT IN SPORT—EXCEPT WHEN IT ISN'T

Anti-doping skeptics make a near-fetish of pointing to modern poles as an example of sport embracing technology that enhances performance. Norman Fost, an early and persistent critic we encountered earlier, wrote: "The use of a fiberglass pole instead of a bamboo pole by pole-vaulters was initially resisted because of the obvious advantage it gave to those who had it. The response was not to ban it, but to make it available to everyone. This produced a different sport, perhaps less natural than its predecessor, but not one that is inherently immoral."[12] [(p7)]

Fost is mistaken about both the history of pole vaulting and about the reasons why the sport acted as it did. Aluminum, steel, and fiberglass poles had been permitted for more than a decade before vaulters began setting records with fiberglass poles. More important is his assumption that fiberglass was resisted because it was "unnatural." But it wasn't resisted, any more than other unnatural materials such as aluminum and steel. "Naturalness" had nothing to do with what was acceptable in pole vaulting. A.C. Gilbert, the "hatchet man" of the 1908 London Olympics, encountered far more resistance from the rulers of sport than did fiberglass pole pioneers. It's true that Bob Seagren failed to win gold at the 1972 Munich Olympics when he was forbidden to use his innovative "Cata-pole" on the grounds that his competitors didn't have one; but they were using "old-fashioned" fiberglass! So the issue has nothing to do with unnaturalness. The claimed rationale—however flimsy—for denying Seagren the right to use the pole he'd trained on was fairness: that his pole, which may have been a superior technology, was not available to his competitors. This, of course, was the same argument offered by speed skaters unable to get their hands on the best klapskates.

Consider Fost's claim that it shouldn't matter whether the means for enhancing performance are natural or not. He has a point. We don't much care if a runner wears a jersey and shorts made from "natural" cotton or wool or from synthetic fibers. We don't insist that her shoes be fashioned from leather alone; exotic combinations of natural and synthetic materials are fine. Wood and bamboo poles may be more "natural" than steel, aluminum or fiberglass, but so what? Fost is right so far. But he leaps from this unexceptional observation to a strange conclusion: that fiberglass poles made vaulting a "different sport . . . less natural than its predecessor . . ."

How would we know whether we'd created a "different" sport? Vaulters were leaping higher, that's for sure. (Just as they'd done using natural bamboo rather than stiff, equally natural wooden poles.) But they were running down the same track, planting their poles in the same boxes, following the same rules. And, most important, the most gifted, hardest-working athletes were still winning. Speed, strength, and tallness—Ganslen's criteria for greatness in the pole vault—were what made the difference between winners and also-rans.

Fost confuses the naturalness of external factors—in this case, what the pole was made from—with the kind of naturalness that matters to sport: the natural talents that each athlete brings to the competition. Wisdom in sport requires understanding when to welcome innovation and when to resist it. Let's say a vaulter showed up with cleverly designed shoes equipped with small downward-facing explosive charges in their soles. The vaulter could detonate them just as he left the ground, giving him a boost upward at the crucial moment. I am guessing that he'd evoke a response similar to the one A.C. Gilbert's hatchet got from the English in 1908. Except, in this case, the officials would be on much firmer ground. Or, as some transhumanists have suggested, suppose our vaulter had his own body surgically modified—say, a small jet-pack sewn into his back he could fire off to propel him higher than his more gifted, harder-working competitors.[13]

The problem, I've discovered, with absurd hypotheticals such as rocket man is that they often turn out to be true. Femke Van den Driessche, a Belgian cyclocross racer, was found to have a small motor and battery concealed in her bike's seat tube, connected via Bluetooth to a button hidden under the tape covering her handlebar. Very handy if you need a boost up a steep hill. She claimed the bike she was riding belonged to a friend. That didn't convince the disciplinary board hearing her case: She was banned from the sport for six years for "mechanical doping."[14]

Rocket man would also be disqualified, I hope. Not only, as Fost allows, because he has an unfair advantage. Many opponents of anti-doping say the way to eliminate unfairness is to give the technology to everyone. But now we've replaced one problem with two bigger ones. The first problem is the familiar coercive power of performance-enhancing technologies in sport. If jetpacks gave a significant performance boost, and they were permitted, any athlete who wanted to remain competitive would have to undergo the same surgery. That's a nasty choice we shouldn't ask young athletes to make.

The second problem, though, is just as important: the meaning of pole vaulting would be threatened. Success in the vault would have more to do with the skill of surgeons and rocket-builders than with athletes' speed, grace, technique, or dedication.

Performance-enhancing drugs are like a shortcut in the marathon. Runners can reach the finish line faster if they skip a lap and run 20 miles instead of 26 miles, 385 yards. But then they've run a 20-mile race, not a marathon. You could have a game with clubs, balls, a course, and three-foot wide holes, but it wouldn't be golf. As long as we value natural talents along with the virtues required to perfect those talents, then EPO, anabolic steroids, and other performance-enhancing drugs undermine those values and distort the meanings we seek in sport.

The line between "natural" and "unnatural" can be tough to see at times, but just because boundaries are difficult to draw doesn't make them useless. The vistas afforded by the Grand Canyon and Disney World may both have their appeal. But we can still appreciate that the Grand Canyon's beauty is natural in a way Disney World's manufactured and manicured prettiness is not. If a movement ever arises to preserve Disney World, it's likely to come from very different motivations—preservation of a particular era in American popular entertainment—than what stirs people to protect the Grand Canyon, Yellowstone, and Muir Woods. When we emphasize something's naturalness, we are pointing at what we believe is a source of its value.

The achievements of athletes, from the fumbling beginner to the most polished Olympian or pro, find their meaning and value in the celebration of whatever natural talents those persons bring to their sport, and how well they perfect those talents.

NOTES

1. Burke MD, Roberts TJ. Drugs in sport: An issue of morality or sentimentality. *J Philos Sport*. 1997;24(1):99–113.
2. van Hilvoorde I, Vos R, de Wert G. Flopping, klapping, and gene doping: Dichotomies between "natural" and "artificial" in elite sports. *Soc Stud Sci*. 2007;37:173–200.

3. Versteeg R. Arresting vaulting pole technology. *Vanderbilt J Entertain Tech Law.* 2005;8(1):93–117.

4. Ganslen RV. *Mechanics of the pole vault.* St. Louis, MO: John Swift; 1973. 167 p.

5. O'Connor LM, Vozenilek JA. Is it the athlete or the equipment? An analysis of the top swim performances from 1990 to 2010. *J Strength Cond Res Natl Strength Cond Assoc.* 2011 Dec;25(12):3239–3241.

6. Barrow JD. Why ban full-body Olympics swimsuits? A scientist explains polyurethane [Internet]. *The Daily Beast.* 2012 Jul 25 [cited 2016 Apr 21]. Available from: http://www.thedailybeast.com/articles/2012/07/25/why-ban-full-body-olympics-swimsuits-a-scientist-explains-polyurethane.html.

7. Crouse K. Faster racing suits may soon be banned from competition. *New York Times* [Internet]. 2009 May 18 [cited 2016 Dec 30]. Available from: http://www.nytimes.com/2009/05/18/sports/othersports/18swim.html.

8. Loland S, Murray TH. The ethics of the use of technologically constructed high-altitude environments to enhance performances in sport. *Scand J Med Sci Sports.* 2007 Jun;17(3):193–193.

9. Halberstam D. *The Breaks of the Game.* New York: Hyperion; 2009. 416 p.

10. Rawls J. Letter to Owen Fiss [Internet]. *The Boston Review.* 1981 [cited 2016 Dec 29]. Available from: http://bostonreview.net/rawls-the-best-of-all-games.

11. Simon RL. *The Ethics of Sport: What Everyone Needs to Know.* New York: Oxford University Press; 2016. 264 p.

12. Fost N. Banning drugs in sports: A skeptical view. *The Hastings Center Report.* 1986;16(4):5–10.

13. Miah A. Enhanced athletes? It's only natural [Internet]. *The Washington Post.* 2008 Aug 3. [cited 2016 Dec 28]. Available from: http://www.washingtonpost.com/wp-dyn/content/article/2008/08/01/AR2008080103060.html.

14. VeloNews. Van den Driessche banned six years for hidden motor [Internet]. *VeloNews.com.* 2016 Apr 26. [cited 2016 Jul 27]. Available from: http://velonews.competitor.com/2016/04/news/van-den-driessche-banned-six-years-for-hidden-motor_403450.

Chapter 4

What's Fair? Aristotle, the Paralympics, and the Pursuit of Excellence

For if some be slow, and others swift, that is no reason why the one should have little and the others much; it is in gymnastic contests that such excellence is rewarded.

Aristotle, *Politics*

The 100-meter Olympic sprint requires explosive acceleration, great form, and the stamina not to fade in the final meters. Usain Bolt won gold along with the unofficial title "fastest man in the world" when he won the event at the 2012 London Games. Shelly-Ann Fraser-Pryce, known as the "pocket rocket," won the women's 100-meter race. That makes a grand total of two gold medals in the 100 meters, the same number as in 1928, the first year women were allowed to compete in Olympic track and field events. An American high school student, Betty Robinson, won gold that year with a world-record time of 12.2 seconds.

In the 2016 Rio Paralympic Games, thirty finals were run in the same 100-meter event: sixteen for men, fourteen for women. The number has varied over the years as classification schemes have been redrawn and the numbers of elite athletes within each category has fluctuated. For male Paralympians in 2016, three separate finals took place for athletes with different degrees of visual impairment; six for different levels of "coordination impairment" caused by, for example, cerebral palsy or traumatic brain injury; three for "limb deficiencies" such as amputations; and four for wheelchair athletes who must compete seated because of loss of function in the lower limbs. Women competed in all of the same categories as men except for T51, the most severe level of spinal cord injury, and T33, with impairments such as those resulting from cerebral palsy or traumatic brain injuries.[1]

Why so many? The short answer is to keep the competition interesting, fair, and meaningful. Interesting, because a match between vastly unequal athletes would not be competitive: We'd know the winner far in advance. Fair, because athletes want to compete on a "level playing field." Meaningful in that the outcome is determined by what we believe should separate winners from losers. The "level playing field" cannot and should not eliminate all differences among athletes, only those that get in the way of what gives the event its meaning and value. Assuring that the playing field is level enough requires making two sorts of judgments. First, we must decide which of all possible differences ought to count in determining who wins and who loses. Second, we have to sort athletes into eligibility groups that allow the factors identified in that first decision to come to the fore.

In a sports competition, as in any situation in which rewards are distributed unequally, abiding by fairness requires choosing which factors should be allowed to make a difference and which should not. The Olympics were born in ancient Greece, as was philosophy, which meant, simply, love of wisdom. The great philosopher Aristotle provided a description of fairness for the ages: Treat like cases alike, and different cases differently. Hard to argue with Aristotle, especially when he makes such good sense. But, of course, everything hangs on what makes cases alike, and what makes them different—a question the Paralympics has had to face more often and more directly than most sport organizations.

Make no mistake: Today's Paralympians are elite athletes, driven to excel. Ludwig Guttmann, a visionary physician, wanted to revolutionize the treatment of people with spinal cord injuries like the former servicemen and women in his care at the Stoke Mandeville Hospital. Competitive sport, he believed, would help their bodies recover strength and coordination; it also would give them a sense of purpose and a meaningful future in society. What began as an archery competition between severely paralyzed patients at two hospitals in England in 1948 has grown into a formidable international movement featuring extraordinary athletes with a wide range of impairments.[2] Paralympic competitions are as intensely competitive as the Olympic Games. The International Paralympic Committee's vision statement begins: "To Enable Paralympic Athletes to Achieve Sporting Excellence and Inspire and Excite the World." For this vision to be meaningful, we need a clear conception of what "sporting excellence" is. And we need to be able to stage competitions that allow sporting excellence to be displayed and rewarded.

Of course, the playing field is never perfectly level. Some athletes will have better coaches than others, better equipment, access to top-quality training facilities and the expertise of sports scientists. Some will be more dedicated and work harder. And, finally, some athletes will simply be more talented than their competitors. Resources, opportunities, dedication, and talent—all these provide relative advantages or disadvantages to each competitor. The first two—resources and opportunities— tilt the field away from ideal fairness. The Paralympic movement is under constant pressure to reduce disparities between athletes from rich and poor nations in access to equipment such as racing wheelchairs. More on that in a moment.

Fairness in sport commands attention. Hitters in baseball know right away when an umpire is calling a wider strike zone for the other team's pitcher than for their own. Basketball players are always on the lookout for referees whose calls favor their opponents. When the people officiating a game enforce the rules unevenly, every player and every fan understands that's unfair. Imagine the reaction in a football game if one of the teams were forced to use a heavy, misshapen ball while the other team was given an elegant standard issue one when it went on offense. Unfair! Or, to take a recent case, one team uses partially deflated footballs that are easier to grip.

You don't need to be an expert on sports to understand that games need to be fair, that both teams need to play under the same rules, that the rules need to be evenly enforced, and that the conditions of play must not place one team at a notable disadvantage. That's why games such as soccer, football, and basketball change sides of the pitch, field, or court halfway through. If wind, or condition of the turf, or softness of a rim favors teams playing on that side for the first half, the other team gets that advantage for the remainder of the contest. These are common ways sport tries to ensure fairness. The challenge is especially tough with Paralympic athletes.

CLASSIFICATION

How do you create a fair, level playing field for Paralympic competitors with no fewer than ten different categories of impairment: in vision; strength; range of movement; limb deficiency; leg length difference; hypertonia; ataxia (problems with

coordination, movement, and balance); athetosis (slow, writh-
ing, involuntary movements); short stature; and intellectual
impairment? Not only that, but within each major type there can
be notable variations in the degree of impairment. If that's not
complicated enough, consider that the same impairment may
have different consequences for an athlete's performance in different sports. Each sport is tasked with justifying how it groups
athletes for competition. In 2009 the International Paralympic
Committee (IPC) published a "Position Stand" on the science and
context of classification in Paralympic sport. The goal, it affirms,
is: " . . . all Paralympic systems of classification should indicate
that the purpose of the system is to promote participation in
sport by people with disabilities by minimising the impact of eligible types of impairment on the outcome of competition."[3] (p19)

Track and field, known collectively as athletics, provides no
fewer than forty-nine classes for competition: sixteen for running and jumping events, seven for wheelchair racing, fifteen
for standing throws, and eleven for seated throws. If cerebral
palsy is the reason you need a wheelchair, you will be assigned
to one of three classes depending on how much your coordination is impaired, your arm and trunk strength, and your grasp.
If instead your impairment comes from an injured spinal cord
or an amputation, four classifications are possible up to athletes
with full muscle power in their arms and trunk who receive a T54
classification. Pitting someone rated T54 against other athletes
with no power from their trunk muscles, diminished shoulder
muscles, and who cannot easily straighten their elbows to push
the chair's wheels (the criteria for T51) would be meaningless.
The impairment's severity would be decisive, not the athletes' talents and dedication.

Fair enough. Impairment, by itself, shouldn't determine
who wins or loses. Parathletes should compete against other

parathletes whose impairments have a comparable impact on their performance. Sometimes impairments array themselves into rough natural categories. People with above-the-knee amputations have more difficulty running than people with below-the-knee amputations. So it wouldn't be fair to the above-the-knee parathlete to be forced to run against below-the-knee competitors. But many lines are difficult to draw. The IPC offers this counsel: "Given that classes must always span a range of activity limitation, the most important guiding principle for setting the number of classes should be that within any given class, the range of activity limitation should never be so large that athletes with impairments causing the greatest activity limitation are significantly disadvantaged when competing against those with impairments causing the least activity limitation."[3 (p30)]

If the degree of activity limitation *shouldn't* be allowed to determine who wins or loses, what ought to make the decisive difference? Paralympic classification schemes face a clarifying challenge: Should an athlete be classified strictly according to their current abilities or to their impairments? Here's the problem: Athletes who have trained diligently and suffered for their sport may present with a comparable level of strength as other athletes with lesser impairments, but who have, shall we say, a more relaxed idea of preparation. On certain measures of strength directly related to performance, they may be equal because the athlete with more severe impairments has worked so much harder.

This looks like a clear injustice. If dedication is one of those factors in Aristotle's formula as applied to sport that makes cases unlike, we shouldn't penalize it. What makes the playing field level is the underlying impairment, not the individual's current ability. The hardest-working, most talented athlete should prevail. It would be helpful if we could gauge impairment without discriminating against the most dedicated athletes. One proposal is to measure isometric strength rather than power. Parathletes typically train to increase power, not isometric strength, so measuring isometric strength is a more direct index of the underlying impairment. Wrestling with such questions is a never-ending challenge for parathletes and the people who work with them to stage fair and meaningful competitions.[4]

The task of fair classification is complex. For one thing, parasport scientists caution that "each Paralympic sport should identify those activities that are fundamental to performance in that sport, and then operationally describe criteria for each eligible impairment type that will impact on the execution of those fundamental activities."[3 (p22)] It's no surprise that decisions about what counts as more or less equivalent impairments, and how to assess them accurately, continue to be debated.[5]

And then, of course, there's cheating. Tweedy and Vanlandewijck cite anecdotal evidence that athletes occasionally misrepresent their level of impairment hoping to get a more favorable classification. The Paralympic movement takes this possibility very seriously. Violators can be banned for life. In the run-up to the 2016 Paralympic Games in Rio, the IPC reviewed more than eighty allegations of intentional misrepresentation. None of them, the IPC concluded, reached the required standard of proof, though a number of athletes were referred for reassessment.[6] Britain's Baroness Grey-Thompson, an eleven-time Paralympic champion, said the issue "goes to the heart of the integrity of the sport."[7]

The most notorious case of intentional misrepresentation in the Paralympics was Spain's "intellectually impaired" basketball team in the 2000 Paralympic Games. Morally impaired is more like it. Ten of the twelve team members had no intellectual impairment. The hoax was exposed when Carlos Ribagorda, a journalist who had played for the Spanish squad, alerted the IPC and made the scandal public.[8]

"Boosting" is another form of cheating. Athletes with spinal cord injuries have been known to stress their bodies—sitting on thumbtacks is one method—to raise their blood pressure and heart rate. An elevated heart rate enhances performance. The IPC prohibits boosting; officials can monitor blood pressure and, if it's high, make the athlete wait until it returns to the normal range.[9,10]

How refined must classifications be? Consider the recommendations made in a discussion paper submitted to an IPC Athletics Summit.[11] The panel of more than twenty experts recommended changing the eligibility for runners with unilateral upper limb amputations from through or above the wrist to through or above the elbow. Why? Because below-elbow amputations don't have much of an effect on the ability to run or to throw (assuming that the throwing is done with the intact arm, of course). The impact on straight line running of losing an entire forearm, though small, is enough to affect the outcome of a race. The panel also examined the evidence as to whether starting from a crouch (which would be more difficult for a person with only one hand) was a notable advantage over a standing start. Not enough, they concluded, to justify a separate classification.

The need for practical wisdom was never more visible than in the panel's analysis of bend running. What's bend running? In events longer than 100 meters, athletes have to navigate curves. Runners are always going counter-clockwise around the track, leaning to their left into the curves and pumping hard with their right arms. Losing all or part of your right arm would be a disadvantage in the 200-meter and 400-meter events because athletes are navigating a curved track, going all-out for the full race.

In longer races, speeds are slower and the impact of a unilateral amputation is less important.

The panel noted that "right-arm amputation will have a much bigger impact on bend running than left-arm amputation, but there has never been any suggestion that right arm amputees should compete in a different class from left-arm amputees, or that right-arm amputees should be eligible for bend running events, and left-arm amputees should not be . . . "[11 (p1–2)]

Are runners who lost their right arms at a competitive disadvantage in the 200-meter and 400-meter races to runners who lost their left arms? The panel seems to think so. Is that a good enough reason to create separate events according to which arm you lost? No, they concluded. The point isn't to create a perfectly level playing field, just a reasonably fair one. The apotheosis of the perfectly level playing field is one on which a single unique athlete performs. After all, no two people are exactly alike.

TECHNOLOGY AS ENABLING VERSUS ENHANCING

There would be no pole-vaulting without poles and crossbars, and no wheelchair races without racing wheelchairs. Many Paralympic events could not take place without technology. For the discus, javelin, and shot put, athletes in wheelchairs need special frames that stabilize their bodies while they throw. Runners with visual impairments need tethers connecting them to a sighted partner who can help them remain on course. The line between technologies that *enable* and technologies that *enhance* can seem thin, but the Paralympic movement takes it very seriously.

Oscar Pistorius achieved fame as the "blade runner" for the J-shaped carbon fiber prostheses he wore in competition. Both of his legs had been amputated below the knee. In the 2008 Paralympic Games, Pistorius won gold in the 100-, 200- and 400-meter events. But he wanted to run in the Olympic Games as well. A dispute ensued over whether his blades gave him an advantage over runners with legs of flesh and bone—whether, that is, his prostheses were a kind of technological enhancement. After the international governing body for athletics, IAAF, ruled that the "Cheetahs" on which Pistorius ran gave him an unfair advantage, he appealed to the Court of Arbitration for Sport, which overturned the IAAF decision and allowed him to compete in the 2012 Olympic Games. He won no medals there, but at the 2012 Summer Paralympic Games, he was chosen to carry the flag in the opening ceremony and went on to win gold medals in the 400-meter event and as a team member in the 4x100 meter relay.

Pistorius was not happy finishing second in the 200-meter event. He accused the winner, Alan Oliveira, of having an unfair technological advantage because his blades were a tad longer than Pistorius's. The IPC's formula for blade length is proportionate to the athlete's estimated body height. Oliveira, being taller, was permitted to use longer blades proportionate to his height. Jerome Singleton, an American competitor in the event, had a different complaint. Singleton was a single amputee unlike Oliveira and Pistorius, both double amputees. Singleton argued that it was unfair to make people like him race against runners on two blades. (Singleton's complaint is consistent with the IAAF's initial judgment that the blades are, on the whole, an enhancing technology.)

Pistorius's fame turned to infamy when in 2013 he shot and killed his girlfriend, Reeva Steenkamp, at his home in Pretoria. He claimed that he thought he was shooting at an intruder. Charged with murder, Pistorius was initially found guilty of a lesser charge—culpable homicide. Prosecutors' appeal was heard before a five-judge panel of the Supreme Court of Appeals. By a unanimous vote, the panel overturned the culpable homicide conviction and found him guilty of murder. At this writing, he is serving a six-year sentence.

The Paralympic movement's confrontation with Aristotle's challenge is also visible in its rulings on new equipment. In the 2016–17 Athletics Rules and Regulations, the International Paralympic Committee set out their basic principles. Section 3.3 deals with "Technology and Equipment." The IPC describes four "fundamental principles" it uses to guide "the evolution of equipment": Safety, Fairness, Universality, and Physical Prowess.[12]

Safety isn't difficult to explain or defend, although the IPC's version of it is broader than most. They are concerned for the safety of the athlete, of course, but also of "other competitors, officials, spectators and the environment." If you want spectators and officials around, it's a good idea to avoid equipment likely to impale or cudgel them, so including safety as a fundamental principle is easy enough to justify.

Fairness as a principle brings us closer to the meaning of sport. The IPC adds this explanation: "i.e., the athlete does not receive an unfair advantage that is not within the 'spirit' of the event they are contesting." The scare quotes around "spirit" are a sort of promissory note. The IPC is on to something here: We can't know what's fair or unfair—what to treat as alike or unlike—without understanding what the particular sport is about. It's often true that, as Ecclesiastes reminds us, "under the sun the race is not to the swift, nor the battle to the strong, nor bread to the wise, nor riches to the intelligent, nor favor to the skillful; but time and chance happen to them all" (9:11). The point of creating a "level playing field" in sport is to make it more likely than not that the swift *will* win the race, although time and chance, injury and misfortune, can deprive the swift of victory at any moment. We can't possibly know what's fair without understanding what *ought to* make a difference. Ecclesiastes would have no point to make about time and chance if no one understood that being swift is how you win races.

Aristotle would agree. In his *Politics*, he uses a sport analogy in arguing that offices of state ought to be distributed by merit. (His ideas about what should count as merit may seem foreign to modern sensibilities, to be sure.) He writes: "For if some be slow, and others swift, that is no reason why the one should have little and the others much; it is in gymnastic contests that such excellence is rewarded."[13] (1283:13–14) Yet again, the challenge is to determine what should make cases alike and what should make them different. Politics is one thing; sport, another.

The third principle, Universality, is directed at a particular kind of unfairness. The IPC wants to make certain that technologies are "reasonably commercially available to all." If only athletes from my country can get these fabulous wheelchairs, carbon fiber blades, or whatever technology provides a major advantage, that's not fair to those in other countries. Technology, rather than the athletes' talents and efforts, would be determining the winner.

The fourth and final principle underscores what should matter. That principle is Physical Prowess. The IPC offers this explanation: "human performance is the critical endeavour not the impact of technology and equipment." Explicitly forbidden are "unrealistic enhancements" of height (for throwing events) or stride length. Also prohibited are "materials or devices that store, generate or deliver energy and/or are designed to provide function to enhance performance beyond the natural physical capacity of the athlete."[12] [(Sec. 3.3.2 (1d))] Parathletes are athletes first of all. Paralympic sport values talent and dedication, same as Olympic sport.

With ten distinct categories of impairments, some with multiple degrees of severity, creating level playing fields for Paralympic athletes means paying close attention to values and meanings in sport. Paralympic officials have had to be explicit about the factors that should influence results, and about what counts as a fair competition. Looking at how the Paralympics tries to meet Aristotle's challenge to treat like cases alike and different cases differently underscores the central place of meanings and values in sport. The Paralympics experience also shows the practical and conceptual challenges encountered when you want to create fair and meaningful contests.

Like the Olympics, the Paralympics also bans performance-enhancing drugs despite the complexities of enforcing such a ban when many of its athletes rely on drugs to maintain health or manage symptoms. TUEs (Therapeutic Use Exemptions) are far more common among Paralympians than Olympians. Nevertheless, the Paralympics has an active anti-doping program, and athletes continue to get caught.

If you believe that the "spirit of sport" includes talent and dedication, but not steroids, EPO or other performance-enhancing drugs, you have an obligation to do the best you can to meet Aristotle's challenge by keeping PEDs out of sport. The Paralympics strives to neutralize technological advantages along with differences in impairments so that talent and dedication matter most. Doping is just another technological shortcut that distorts the relationship between what we believe matters in a sport—such as strength, speed, stamina, courage, and dedication—and success in competition.

NOTES

1. International Paralympic Committee. Historical results [Internet]. Available from: https://www.paralympic.org/results/historical.
2. Gold JR, Gold MM. Access for all: The rise of the Paralympic Games. *J R Soc Promot Health*. 2007 May;127(3):133–141.
3. Tweedy SM, Vanlandewijck YC. International Paralympic Committee position stand: Background and scientific principles of classification in Paralympic sport. *Br J Sports Med* [Internet]. 2011 Apr;45(4):259–269. Available from: http://www.ncbi.nlm.nih.gov/pubmed/19850575.
4. Tweedy SM, Williams G, Bourke J. Selecting and modifying methods of manual muscle testing for classification in Paralympic sport. *Eur J Adapt Phys Act*. 2010;3(2):7–16.
5. Howe D. *The Cultural Politics of the Paralympic Movement: Through an Anthropological Lens*. London: Routledge; 2008. 208 p.
6. Silverman I. The IPC's statement related to intentional misrepresentation [Internet]. *SwimSwam*. 2016 Aug 12 [cited 2016 Nov 30]. Available from: https://swimswam.com/ipcs-statement-related-intentional-misrepresentation/.
7. BBC News. Rio Paralympics 2016: Classification is "bedrock" of sport says BPA chief [Internet]. *BBC Sport*. 2016 [cited 2016 Nov 30]. Available from: http://www.bbc.com/sport/disability-sport/37286362.
8. Tremlett G. The cheats. *The Guardian* [Internet]. 2004 Sep 15 [cited 2016 Jul 27]; Available from: https://www.theguardian.com/sport/2004/sep/16/gilestremlett.features11.
9. Collier R. Most Paralympians inspire, but others cheat. *CMAJ Can Med Assoc J*. 2008 Sep;179(6):524.
10. Blauwet CA, Benjamin-Laing H, Stomphorst J, Van de Vliet P, Pit-Grosheide P, Willick SE. Testing for boosting at the Paralympic games: Policies, results and future directions. *Br J Sports Med*. 2013 Sep;47(13):832–837.
11. Tweedy SM, Discussion Paper—Changing the eligibility criterion for unilateral upper limb amputation in IPC Athletics, Presented at IPC Athletics Summit 27.2 – 1.3.2009, Bonn Germany.
12. International Paralympic Committee. International Paralympic Committee Athletics Rules and Regulations 2016–2017. Jan 2016. 2016. Available from: https://www.paralympic.org/sites/default/files/document/160126174701371_2016_01_26+IPC+Athletics+Rules+and+Regulations_A4_Final.pdf.
13. Aristotle. *Politics*. New York: Random House; 1941.

Chapter 5

Inequalities and the Challenge of Creating Fair, Meaningful, and Interesting Competitions

In organized baseball there has been no distinction raised except tacit understanding that a player of Ethiopian descent is ineligible—the wisdom of which we will not discuss except to say that by such a rule some of the greatest ball players the game has ever known have been denied their opportunity.

Unsigned editorial in *The Sporting News*, 6 December 1923

If natural talents, dedication and courage should be the chief difference-makers in sport, what can we make of the host of other factors that lead to success? Many people's talents never get recognized and nurtured simply because their circumstances aren't favorable. For those who get far enough to begin competing there are factors so dominant in certain sports—age, size, and sex—that separate events must be organized. Otherwise, talent, dedication, and courage would be overwhelmed by features we believe shouldn't matter. Sport can never escape Aristotle's challenge; it has to make judgments about what makes athletes alike and what makes them different. And it must set criteria for eligibility for the competitions to be fair, meaningful, and interesting.

THE LEVEL PLAYING FIELD: GEOGRAPHY AND CIRCUMSTANCES

The last chapter opened with Usain Bolt's status as the world's fastest man. He holds that title by virtue of winning the Olympic 100-meter sprint. But we can't really know that he is faster than any other person in the world because so many people never get the opportunity to develop their talents. Is there a superb potential sprinter among the world's 59.5 million forcibly displaced persons? (This includes 19.5 million refugees and almost twice that number classified as "internally displaced persons"—people living in their countries but forced from their homes according to the UN High Commissioner for Refugees.) Or living at home in such desperate poverty that he cannot think about anything but survival? Or perhaps he lives in relative ease but his parents discouraged his pursuit of running, or his coaches failed to recognize and nurture his talents?

People don't succeed as athletes for many reasons. Imagine two identically gifted young women: One has terrific support from family, great coaches, top-quality equipment, time to practice, and the money to get to desirable competitions; the other has none of these. The first athlete has far better opportunities to develop her talents, have them recognized, and move up in the ranks. It will be no surprise if she's more successful in her sport than the equally talented person who lacks these advantages. The two are alike in talent and drive, yet their fates likely will be far different. Is that unfair? If it is, are we obliged to do something to redress that unfairness? Who's responsible, and what should they do?

Geography and climate can make a difference. Most medal winners in the 2010 Vancouver Winter Olympics came from cold places. The top five nations—the United States, Germany, Canada, Norway, and Austria—took more than half of all the medals: 132 out of 258. Notice anything these countries have in common? Try mountains and snow.

In the 2014 Winter Olympics in Sochi, Russia, Norway won eleven gold medals, second only to Russia's thirteen. There is compelling evidence that Russia's sudden climb up the medal count in Sochi was aided by systematic doping, covered up by its anti-doping lab in collusion with Russia's internal intelligence agency, the F.S.B. The lab's director, Grigory Rodchenkov, claims he was told each night which sample bottles to pass through a concealed hole in the wall; the bottles would be returned by morning with the incriminating urine replaced by samples showing no sign of performance-enhancing drugs. According to Rodchenkov, as many as a hundred samples were altered during this operation.[1] He also claimed that at least fifteen of Russia's thirty-three medal winners at Sochi were doping.[2]

Norway is under no comparable cloud, yet with a population of fewer than five million people, Norwegian athletes won twenty-three medals in the 2010 Games including nine golds—as many gold medals as the United States. Norwegian athletes have advantages for winter sports not readily available to athletes in, say, Singapore, Eritrea, or Nicaragua, countries with roughly comparable numbers of residents. Norway is a nation of long, cold winters, mountains, and a cross-country skiing path around its capital city, Oslo. The statue honoring Norway's late king, Olav V, portrays him on cross-country skis. All nine of Norway's gold medals in Vancouver were won on skis, eight in cross-country or biathlon, which combines cross-country skiing with shooting, as were all eleven at Sochi. A child growing up in Norway likely will be encouraged to ski, surrounded by people who love to ski, and, if that child shows talent, to have that talent identified and nurtured. If the same child lived in Singapore, where cross-country skiing simply isn't available as an option, that same talent might be channeled into a different sport in which endurance is a crucial factor.

Climate and geography shape opportunities. They don't strictly determine them. An equatorial country could establish a system to identify children whose physiology seemed favorable for Nordic skiing and ship them off to cold mountainous climes for training. It's a good thing they generally don't. The disruption in children's and families' lives caused by being sent to a foreign place to live among strangers is a high price to pay to satisfy a nation's ambition for Olympic medals.

The sources of disadvantage are much broader than just climate and geography. It's not enough to have supportive parents and coaches. Some children born with great natural talents are sidetracked by illness or injury. And by the luck of the biological draw, some never inherited much in the way of athletic ability. These are all sources of difference. When do discrepancies in circumstances become unfair in the context of sport?

FAIRNESS *IN COMPETITION* AND FAIRNESS IN *ACCESS TO COMPETITION*

The distinction between fairness *in competition* on the one hand, and fairness of *access to competition* on the other may be helpful here. Athletes and teams should be treated fairly in competition. Everyone should be governed by the same rules, and those rules should be applied and interpreted without bias. No competitors should have the playing conditions tilted in their favor. Cyclists in the Tour de France, for example, are not allowed to have motors bolted to their bikes, a performance aid that can sound quite appealing to an amateur cyclist laboring up a long steep climb. The notable exceptions to the rule against tilting the playing field, such as golf handicaps, support the general principle. In tournaments that mix golfers of different abilities, less skilled golfers are given a certain number of strokes in order to make a contest that otherwise would be one-sided more interesting. No one pretends that the golfer with a high handicap is a better golfer than one playing without any handicap—a scratch golfer. And in professional tournaments, all golfers play without handicaps.

Norwegian cross-country skiers have advantages over skiers from, say, Ethiopia. That nation's single athlete in the 2010 Vancouver Olympics finished 93rd in the 15-kilometer cross-country freestyle event. No one is claiming that Ethiopia's skier was forced to navigate a different course, use rough planks instead of high-end skis, or was cheated by the officials. Describing a ski trail that goes up and down mountain slopes as "level" seems ludicrous, but the metaphor is clear enough. The contest was fair *in competition*. Geography and other circumstances certainly shape opportunities—what I'm calling fairness in *access to competition*—but to prove that they are morally significant sources of unfairness requires much more. Should we be indignant that Norwegians' success in the Winter Olympics was far out of proportion to its population? That Nicaraguans, Singaporeans, and Eritreans were completely unrepresented at those Games? There are better targets for our moral indignation.

HUMAN RIGHTS AND ANTIDISCRIMINATION

Aristotle insisted that favorable circumstances should not stand in the way of talent and effort when he wrote in *Politics*: "When a number of flute-players are equal in their art, there is no reason why those of them who are better born should have better flutes given to them; for they will not play any better on the flute, and the superior instrument should be reserved for him who is the superior artist."[3] (1282:32-34)

Likewise, many impediments to access to competition are ethically indefensible. For many important purposes, including all of the protections enumerated in the Universal Declaration of Human Rights, the fact that a person was born rich or poor, or in a country with or without snow-covered mountains, would be completely irrelevant. Anyone claiming that they have a right to torture or enslave persons because of where they were born deserves to be condemned for violating bedrock moral principles and international covenants.

Sport has not always treated all athletes the same. Baseball in America had a long history of discriminating against black players. In the 1880s, black athletes such as Bud Fowler could be found on professional teams dominated by white players. By the end of that decade, organized opposition had solidified. The board of baseball's International League in 1887 directed the League Secretary "to approve no more contracts with colored men."[4] Black players already had been busy creating their own leagues. Robert Peterson, in his book *Only the Ball Was White*, describes the realities and significance of life in what was then called the Negro Leagues: "Negro baseball was Josh Gibson standing loose and easy at the plate in Yankee Stadium and hitting the longest home run ever seen in the House that Ruth Built. And it was the touring Brooklyn Colored Giants arriving, broke and hungry, in a small Pennsylvania city where, because of a scheduling mix-up, no game was arranged, and then playing a hastily called game with the local semipros so they could take up a collection for a meal and enough gas to get to the next town. Negro baseball was at once heroic and tawdry, a gladsome thing and a blot on America's conscience."[4] (p15)

It was wrong then to deny the opportunity to compete because of race, as it is wrong today to discriminate against any athlete. The 2014 Olympic Winter Games in Sochi, Russia, were notable not only for the sophisticated efforts to undermine anti-doping; Sochi also was plagued with homophobic incidents and policies.[5] By the end of that year, the Olympic Movement revised its charter to prohibit discrimination on the basis of sexual orientation. The 2016 edition of the Olympic Charter includes seven "Fundamental Principles of Olympism." The sixth principle now reads: "The enjoyment of the rights and freedoms set forth in this Olympic Charter shall be secured without discrimination of any kind, such as race, colour, sex, sexual orientation, language, religion, political or other opinion, national or social origin, property, birth or other status."[6] Any city wishing to host an Olympics from 2022 onward must pledge to disavow all forms of discrimination listed in the Charter. Fair access to competition requires not erecting discriminatory barriers. How to respond to differences in opportunities is another question.

OPPORTUNITY

Think of athletes' ascent to the highest ranks of elite sport as a climb within an inverted funnel. At the wide bottom, a multitude of aspiring athletes are participating. Talented competitors rise to the next level, where the numbers diminish. And so on, level by level, until the most successful reach the narrow, sparsely populated top of the funnel. Within each level, efforts can be made to assure fair, interesting, and meaningful competitions where the factors that ought to make the difference are highlighted and those that should not are minimized. Of course, efforts to neutralize factors that ought not be influential don't always succeed. Sport treats two sources of potential advantage— opportunities and performance-enhancing technologies—in sharply different ways.

Some fortunate athletes get the best coaches, excellent training facilities, and experts in diet and exercise physiology, while their competitors have to make do with mediocre resources and limited expert advice. Because no one regards these differences as integral to the meaning of sport, it would be better if everyone had equal access to comparable resources. Otherwise, sharp inequalities could overwhelm the differences in talent and dedication that ought to matter. In practice, modest inequalities are tolerated, although the higher athletes ascend within the funnel the greater their chance of receiving the support they need to realize their talent. Nevertheless, many elite athletes, even in wealthy countries, struggle to gain support, especially in less glamorous sports. US speed skater Emily Scott needed food stamps while training for the 2014 Sochi Games, while a leading javelin thrower, Cyrus Hosteler, had to rely on food stamps and unemployment benefits while he trained for the Olympics.[7] Hardships such as these surely deter talented athletes who lack the dedication and resourcefulness shown by Scott and Hosteler. It's fair to ask whether a nation that encourages its athletes to aspire to the Olympic Games therefore has an obligation to provide a decent minimum of support for them.

Sport draws much sharper lines when it comes to advantages provided by technologies. Recall the controversy over the Netherlands' monopoly on klapskates and the International Paralympic Committee's insistence that racing wheelchairs and other such devices must be commercially available to all competitors. The IPC's justification for this policy, that "human performance is the critical endeavour, not the impact of technology and equipment," resonates throughout sport. It also helps explain sport's discomfort with technologies of biomedical enhancement—aka doping.

Anti-doping skeptics often claim that differences in climate, geography, and a host of other circumstances are unfair. Some take the next step and argue that because large differences in circumstances can dwarf whatever performance advantages come from drugs, it's therefore silly to worry about doping. Some go further and tout doping as a remedy for unfairness. Disadvantaged athletes, in this scenario, would use drugs or gene doping to compensate for whatever unfavorable circumstances created those disadvantages.

UNEARNED ≠ UNFAIR, BUT ENHANCING OPPORTUNITY IS GOOD ALL THE WAY AROUND

Differences in opportunities, like differences in natural talents, are mostly unearned. But as is the case with natural talents, unearned is not the same as unfair. Sport highlights differences in natural talents, which then answers Aristotle's challenge: Talent makes different cases different in sport competitions. Differences in opportunities, on the other hand, are certainly unfortunate, but sport doesn't typically factor in "opportunity adjustments" the way it subtracts strokes for less skilled golfers. That said, it would be good to reduce the impact of differences in opportunities because they can distort the relationship among talent, dedication, and courage. What can be done to remedy these inequalities of opportunity? Who is responsible for carrying out those remedies?

We have two avenues available here. One is to widen opportunities for people to participate in sport so that variations in circumstances matter less. The other is to resort to doping as a means of compensating for variations in opportunities.

The first option—giving more people a chance to play, discover, and develop whatever talents they have—is good for many reasons. It would help to level out initial differences in access to sport; at the same time it would spread the benefits of playing sport—in health, social development, self-discipline—to more people. There are challenges here. First, many entities from nations to schools, local governments, and sport organizations all have something to contribute, but their efforts likely will be uncoordinated. We can't identify one single party responsible for the larger picture. Second, sport is one among many goods that communities and governments should pursue along with public health, security, national defense, education, and the environment. Tough choices have to be made about dividing available resources among these goods. Finally, we need to be alert to the possibility that youth sport, in particular, can fail to achieve its goals when young people are pushed to value prizewinning over all else and to risk their long-term flourishing through premature specialization, overtraining, or failing to develop interests and talents beyond sport. With those challenges in mind, creating wider opportunities to play sport is an excellent way to lessen the impact of differences in circumstances.

Using doping to compensate for differences in opportunities is another story. Again you have to choose between two paths. If you want to calibrate the doping to match the opportunity deficit, you'll need criteria to quantify that deficit and you will also need to empower some authority to decide who gets biomedical performance enhancement and how much. If creating a doping-entitlement bureaucracy is unappealing, the obvious alternative is to let everyone decide for himself or herself. Such a free-for-all reignites the arms-race-like dynamic that plagued cycling and other sports. Whatever meaning and values we find in sport will be undermined; health risks will increase as athletes are pushed to take more drugs to stay competitive. Yet there may be little impact on the relative rankings of individual competitors as everyone's performance will be boosted.

There is a notable exception to that generalization. Tyler Hamilton's book *The Secret Race* describes how doping can alter our understanding of "natural talent." Hamilton's normal hematocrit was 42. When the UCI decreed that bike racers would be permitted to compete as long as their hematocrit didn't exceed 50, the message was clear: Do whatever is necessary to get yours to 50. For Hamilton that meant a rise of 8 points, which translated to a substantial 19 percent increase. His teammate Marty Jamison's natural level was 48. Using EPO to raise it to 50 meant a gain of only 2 points—4 percent. Both Hamilton and Jamison were able to enhance their endurance by increasing the concentration of red cells in their blood. But in the fun-house mirror world of EPO-saturated bike racing, Hamilton's naturally low hematocrit meant that he could get a much bigger boost once he added EPO in response to an implied invitation to use it.[8]

KEEPING IT INTERESTING AND MEANINGFUL

There are times you realize you have no chance to win. Perhaps you're a talented and dedicated bicycle racer who happens to be fifteen years old. Or fifty years old. The peak years for bike racers tend to be their mid-twenties to mid-thirties. No matter how gifted and hard-working, neither the teenager nor the fifty-year-old stands much of a chance competing against cyclists in their prime. Or pit a 110-pound boxer against an opponent twice that size. Even if they are equally skilled and fit, the smaller fighter likely will lose.

Sports such as cycling recognize that creating meaningful competitions that reward talent and effort requires allowing athletes to compete against other athletes of roughly the same age. So races are staged for under-19 and under-23 riders as well as "masters" cyclists. UCI, the governing body for bicycle racing, includes three categories for older male track racers: 35–44, 45–54, and over 55. Boxing and other "combat" sports such as judo and kickboxing, along with wrestling and weightlifting, set weight ranges for competitors. Men's boxing is organized into ten different weight classifications; women's boxing into three. The point is to stage interesting and meaningful competitions where talent, dedication, and courage can be decisive.

GENDER

Having men compete against men and women against women is such a common way to level the playing field that it may go unnoticed—until Billy Jean King thrashes Bobby Riggs in three straight sets in Houston, Texas, on 20 September, 1973. Their entrances may have been high camp: King was carried in like Cleopatra, held aloft by four well-muscled men dressed as ancient slaves; Riggs was wheeled in by sexy models pulling his rickshaw. But the tennis was serious, and King's flat-out triumph became a rallying point for women in sport.

Or until a Caster Semenya dashes past her female competitors so decisively that both her performance and her masculine appearance raise questions about her gender. Picture yourself at the starting line for the 800-meter race; standing next to the bulging muscles and masculine build of the woman next to you. You might feel that your chances of winning just plummeted. You are, after all, a woman, and women don't get the larger body-building boost of androgenic hormones such as testosterone that men do. But your competitor seems to have a man's build and strength. It feels unfair.

When Semenya burst onto the world athletic scene as a teen-ager from South Africa, she dominated her competitors in the 800 meters, including an astonishing time of 1:55:45 in the 2009 World Championships in Berlin, fast enough for a gold medal and the prize money that comes with it. Semenya is broad-shouldered with well-defined muscles. But so are many other female athletes. She had shown sudden, dramatic improvements in performance—often a telltale sign of doping. It did not help to dampen suspicion that the head coach of the South African team, Dr. Ekkart Arbeit, had admitted his involvement in the East German doping machine to a German parliamentary inquiry.[9],[10] Arbeit was a Stasi spy for twenty years; Dr. Werner Franke, who with his wife Brigitte Berendonk exposed the depths of East Germany's doping machine, says that Arbeit was responsible for giving steroids to minors.[11] Reportedly, Semenya's medical evaluation showed an extraordinarily high level of testosterone for a woman. The results have not been made public.

In almost every sport, elite men consistently show a signifi-cant performance advantage over elite women. In any given year, the top performance by a woman likely wouldn't crack the top five hundred performances by men in the same event. If women were forced to line up against men of comparable levels of train-ing and skill, a man would win nearly every time. It would be understandable if women out of complete frustration decided to stop competing. Or maybe they'd set up their own events, bar-ring men from competing.

Wait. That's exactly what we have: separate competitions for men and women.

Which is why rare athletes such as Semenya pose a quandary for sport. Gender, we now understand, is a conceptual binary imposed upon nature's continuum. Most humans fit comfortably enough into one of the two categories—but some people don't. Sport has mostly seen this as the challenge of preventing men from masquerading as women. But the line between male and female is not always sharp and clear. Sport is struggling to find a fair and respectful way of allowing all athletes to compete on a more or less level playing field.

How can sport accommodate the biological complexities of gender identity with the performance advantages provided by masculinizing hormones and the desire to stage fair, interesting, and meaningful competitions for *all* women? Coming to terms with this challenge requires exploring the biology of gender, the values of sport, and the legal system for arbitrating disputes in sport. These strands have come together in the story of Dutee Chand, a young Indian runner whose case very likely affected the outcome of the women's 800-meter competition in the Rio Olympics.

NOTES

1. McLaren RH. The independent person report. [Internet]. 2016 Jul 16. Available from: https://www.wada-ama.org/sites/default/files/resources/files/20160718_ip_report_newfinal.pdf.
2. Ruiz RR, Schwirtz, M. Russian insider says state-run doping fueled Olympic gold. *New York Times*. 2016 May 12. [Internet]. Available from: http://www.nytimes.com/2016/05/13/sports/russia-doping-sochi-olympics-2014.html (Accessed 2016 May 24).
3. Aristotle, *Politics*. New York: Random House; 1941.
4. Peterson R. *Only the Ball Was White: A History of Legendary Black Players and All-Black Professional Teams*. Oxford: Oxford University Press; 1992.

5. Rhodan M. Olympic committee adds anti-discrimination clause for host cities. *Time*. 2014 Sept 24. Available from: http://time.com/3427596/olympic-committee-host-discrimination/ (Accessed 2016 Nov 27).

6. International Olympic Committee. Olympic Charter. [Internet]. 2016. Available from: https://stillmed.olympic.org/media/Document%20Library/OlympicOrg/General/EN-Olympic-Charter.pdf (Accessed 2016 Nov 27).

7. Hobson W. 2016. Olympic executives cash in on a "Movement" that keeps athletes poor [Internet]. *The Washington Post*. 2016 Jul 30. Available from: https://www.washingtonpost.com/sports/olympics/olympic-executives-cash-in-on-a-movement-that-keeps-athletes-poor/2016/07/30/ed18c206-5346-11e6-88eb-7dda4e2f2aec_story.html (Accessed 2016 Aug 8).

8. Coyle D, Hamilton T. *The Secret Race: Inside the Hidden World of the Tour de France: Doping, Cover-ups, and Winning at All Costs*. New York: Bantam; 2012.

9. Vinton N. Former East German track coach Ekkart Arbeit caught up in Caster Semenya gender controversy [Internet]. *NY Daily News*. 2009 Aug 25. Available from: http://www.nydailynews.com/sports/more-sports/east-german-track-coach-ekkart-arbeit-caught-caster-semenya-gender-controversy-article-1.397564 (Accessed 2016 Jul 28).

10. Hoberman J. *Testosterone Dreams: Rejuvenation, Aphrodisia, Doping*. Berkeley: University of California Press; 2005.

11. Hoberman J. How drug testing fails: The politics of doping control. In: Wilson W, Derse E, editors. *Doping in Elite Sport: The Politics of Drugs in the Olympic Movement*. New York: Human Kinetics; 2001. p. 241–270.

Chapter 6

Gender, Fairness, and Meaning

(M)ost of us just feel that we are literally running against
a man.

Diane Cummins

Most of the variations in human sexual development are of no
special concern to sport. They matter only when they affect fairness and meaning—when, for example, women are forced to
compete against athletes with the biological advantages common
to men. In such cases, those mismatches threaten to undermine
the connection between natural talents, dedication, and success
that sport values so highly.

By far the most common challenges are athletes who identify
as women but whose bodies show the unmistakable imprint of
large doses of testosterone. Some of these athletes have the pair
of X chromosomes that are the hallmark of genetic femaleness,
but for some reason—a genetic abnormality such as congenital
adrenal hyperplasia, Cushing syndrome, polycystic ovarian syndrome, or a tumor—produce extra testosterone. Other athletes
have the typical male complement of an X and a Y chromosome
but don't experience the full androgenic impact of testosterone.
Partial androgen insensitivity, in which testosterone's masculinizing call is only partly heeded, and 5 alpha reductase deficiency,
in which an enzyme needed to convert testosterone into a related
hormone, DHT, crucial to normal male sexual development, is

missing, likewise can result in a female gender identity but also in strength more typical of men.

Whatever triggered IAAF's investigation of Caster Semenya, it set off an international display of ugliness. Somehow, early details of the inquiry got out—there were reports of a fax getting into the hands of the wrong person. The IAAF declined to talk about the details of its investigation or Semenya's condition. The circus had come to town anyway. An Australian newspaper reporting that Semenya was a hermaphrodite, and a variety of claims about her supposed intersex diagnosis ricocheted around the world.[1]

South Africa's sports establishment outperformed its rivals in the race to the bottom. The Sport Minister warned of a "third world war" if Semenya were not allowed to compete. Complaints of racism were tossed casually around like stink bombs. Athletics South Africa, or ASA, that nation's governing body for track and field, behaved particularly badly. Its president, Leonard Chuene, complained loudly and repeatedly about the unfairness and insensitivity the IAAF was showing toward Semenya. Then it was discovered the ASA had performed its own gender verification tests, despite Chuene's repeated denials. He was suspended along with the rest of the ASA Board, on 5 November 2010.[1]

Some of the women who'd raced against Semenya wanted more information. Diane Cummins, a Canadian runner, asked: " . . . is she a man, is she a lady? What constitutes male, what constitutes female? Even if she is a female, she's on the very fringe of the normal athlete female biological composition from what I understand of hormone testing. So, from that perspective, most of us just feel that we are literally running against a man."[2]

By July 2010, Semenya was once again declared eligible to race as a woman.[3] Eleven months would have been sufficient time for medical interventions that would bring her testosterone levels down to something like those of her competitors. Additional evidence that something had changed was her performance. Until a recent change in policy, she had not come close to matching her time of 1:55.45 in the 2009 World Championships. In a number of races she had taken more than two minutes. She also ran the 1,500 meters, and there her time was five seconds slower following her hiatus from competition. Now, these "slower" times managed to win races in Finland and South Africa. But she didn't win every race: She finished third in the Diamond League event in Brussels less than two months after her return. She continued to improve through the 2012 London Olympics, finishing second with a time of 1:56:19. The runner who beat her, Mariya Savinova, has since been given a lifetime ban for doping.

A DISGRACEFUL HISTORY

Any honest discussion of gender and sport must begin by acknowledging that for most of the modern era, the treatment of women athletes suspected of being men in disguise has been appalling. We now understand that not every person's gender fits neatly into one of two buckets—male or female. It's more realistic to think of gender identity as a continuum. Many factors affect an individual's identity including a variety of medical syndromes classified as DSDs—disorders of sexual development. (Some advocates prefer the phrase *differences* of sexual development.) But neither can we forget that in most sports—those for which size, power or strength is decisive—men have an advantage over women. In those sports where testosterone matters, elite female athletes would have little success competing against elite male athletes.

The quandary is clear: If athletes benefiting significantly from the advantages provided by male levels of testosterone are allowed to compete against women who don't have that advantage, the latter's chances of success shrink. At the same time, women with such conditions deserve respect, including the opportunity to participate in sport. The challenge is to treat all women fairly. Before we look at how we might accomplish this with compassion and wisdom, consider some examples of how to do it really, really badly.

HOW *NOT* TO DEAL WITH GENDER IN SPORT

An injustice shrouded by a lie, drowning in a sea of shame: This is a fair description of what happened to Maria José Martínez-Patiño at the World University Games in Kobe, Japan in 1985. Now Dr. Martínez-Patiño, she owned Spain's national record in the 60-meter hurdles. The day prior to her race she reported, as instructed, to "Sex Control," where cells were scraped from the inside of her cheek—a procedure called a buccal smear. Within hours, she was informed that her test was abnormal. The next day she learned that she'd been disqualified: She had failed her "sex" test.

Martínez-Patiño's cells had both an X and a Y chromosome. Thus, early in her fetal life, testes appeared and began pumping out testosterone, the hormone that directs the body toward the masculine form. But she also inherited a genetic mutation in the androgen receptor gene, located on the X chromosome, leaving her cells deaf to testosterone's masculinizing call, a condition known as androgen insensitivity syndrome (AIS). Unless our tissues and organs heed testosterone's message, our developmental wiring takes the path toward femininity. AIS forms a spectrum ranging from a complete inability to respond to testosterone to a variety of incomplete forms. Complete AIS, as in Martínez-Patiño's case, occurs as often as once in every 20,000 births. More than 150 mutations that can cause AIS have been discovered.

Most people who identify as women inherit a pair of X chromosomes but no Y chromosome. Navigating the path toward maleness requires two components: certain genes on the Y chromosome, which XX females won't have; and well-functioning androgen receptors. If either piece is missing, the fetus will take the path toward developing as a female. Martínez-Patiño, like other XY women with complete AIS, was unquestionably female. The testosterone oozing from her fetal testes found no response so her body took on an unmistakably feminine form. Her biology could deny fertility: Without ovaries, she could produce no eggs. It was human ignorance, though, that denied her the right to participate in the sport she loved and in which she excelled.

Martínez-Patiño was not allowed to compete as a woman in the World University Games. The Spanish sports federation doctor and officials overseeing the Games advised her to fake an injury rather than reveal her "secret." She cried, and had to spend the next week in Japan watching "other girls run my race."[4] She describes sitting in her room, "feeling a sadness that I could not share."[5] Media coverage in Spain and elsewhere asserted that, in Martínez-Patiño's own words, "the 100-meter specialist from Spain was really a 'man,'" amplifying the emotional impact on her and her family. In the weeks and months that followed, Martínez-Patiño wrote, "I lost everything that I had, my athletic scholarship, I had to leave my studies, I lost my friends, my boyfriend, I had to leave my apartment provided for me as an athlete. But the worst suffering was that of knowing that my womanhood was questioned by the whole world."[6]

Confirmed outright frauds—men claiming to be women—are rare or nonexistent. I was unable to find a single confirmed case. "Dora" Ratjen reportedly claimed that the Nazi Youth Movement forced him to disguise himself as a woman, and he finished fourth in the high jump at the 1936 Berlin Olympic Games. But there are credible reports that "Dora," later known as Heinrich, was raised as a girl on the advice of health professionals who had examined him as an infant. It has been reported that he had a penis of some kind, though deformed. On 21 September 1938 at age 19, Ratjen was arrested at the Magdeburg station when Detective Sergeant Sömmering was alerted to the possibility that a man on the train was dressed as a woman. Initially Ratjen refused to cooperate but soon acknowledged he was a man. Ratjen's arrest and identification as a man threw the Reich Sports Ministry into a tizzy. He was sent for further testing to Hohenlychen sports sanatorium, which agreed that he was a man. Threats of criminal prosecution were later dropped, as authorities concluded he had not sought any financial gain from competing as a woman. His medals were returned, and according to *Der Speigel*, he went back to his hometown to work in the bar his parents owned.[7]

Later, the Press sisters, Irina and Tamara, competed for the USSR and dominated their field events through 1965, setting 26 world records and winning six Olympic gold medals. Stocky and muscular, they were suspected of being men masquerading as women. Their failure to appear for a so-called nude parade before a panel of gynecologists in the 1966 European Track and Field Championships in Budapest was widely viewed at the time as confirmation that they were men. More likely, they manifested some form of DSD. Perhaps they feared public exposure and humiliation before a world that would not understand that their difference was a part of natural biological variation. Nearly half a century ago, when the Press sisters and four other women declined to participate in the "nude parade," the social stigma would have been severe.

The nude parade was quickly replaced by a genetic screening test—the buccal smear that led to such grief for Maria José Martínez-Patiño. That test was widely criticized as technically difficult, unreliable, and likely to lead to misclassifications. A person whose tissues cannot respond to the call of testosterone, as Martínez-Patiño's could not, will develop a woman's proportions, breasts, genitalia, and secondary sexual characteristics. A person with complete androgen insensitivity who tried to cheat by taking testosterone would fail: Her body would simply ignore it. Martínez-Patiño is, in all matters relevant to fair competition, a woman just like other women. She should never have been disqualified.

Martínez-Patiño persevered, and in 1988, her eligibility to compete as a woman was restored. She missed qualifying for the 1992 Barcelona Olympics by a tenth of a second. It was not the neat ending she and those who believed in her may have hoped for; but her courage, and the persistence of scientists who championed her cause, such as the Finnish geneticist Albert de la Chapelle and the Swede Arne Lundqvist, rescued a measure of dignity and justice.

What happened to Martínez-Patiño in Kobe was an injustice that began with a faulty understanding of human sexual development and the relationship between her particular disorder—AIS—and athletic performance. Two other women out of the 523 female athletes tested in Kobe in 1985 were disqualified; one of them, like Martínez-Patiño, had AIS.[8] By the 1996 Atlanta Olympics, the IOC was using a more sophisticated analytic technique, polymerase chain reaction—or PCR, which uses tiny bits of DNA to make many copies of itself until there's enough to analyze. Seven of the eight female athletes picked up with this test also had AIS. The eighth had a rare DSD; all eight were permitted to compete as women.[9],[10] The shiny new PCR test proved to be far from infallible. It reliably detects the presence of a Y chromosome—but not whether or how much a performance boost the athlete receives.

By 1999, the IOC's Athletes Commission was calling for an end to routine sex testing; their plea was heeded in time for the 2000 Sydney Summer Games. Olympic Federations followed suit, with Volleyball as the last in 2004. While routine testing ended, organizers were expected to have on hand a team of experts in the event an athlete whose eligibility to compete as a woman appeared in doubt.[11]

A challenge remains in dealing with the rare cases of intersex that may provide a competitive advantage. Unlike Martínez-Patiño, some women may incorporate enough of a man's strength and size to give a significant competitive edge over other women. Sport must be fair to women with such advantages, and also to the women they're competing against.

A SHIFT FROM GENDER
TO HYPERANDROGENISM

Sport has tried to strike a balance between these concerns. On 12 April 2011, the IAAF became the first Olympic body to announce a new policy intended to ensure that women are able to compete fairly against other women. Rather than the diffuse focus on gender verification that blighted earlier attempts to ensure fairness for women athletes, the new policy homes in on the presumed primary source of unfairness: those rare cases in which women produce androgenic hormones such as testosterone at the levels seen in men *and* have tissues that respond to testosterone's muscle-building call. Under the policy, the eligibility of women to compete would be evaluated only if their testosterone levels were ten nanomoles per liter or more—within the normal range for males, and well above the normal range for women.[12] The proposed policy was intended to provide a sensitive, case-by-case evaluation aimed at protecting each athlete's privacy while promoting fair competition for all women. But it has not satisfied everyone, as the case of Dutee Chand made clear.

Chand was born in Chaka Gopalpur village in Odisha, India, on 3 February 1996. By 2007, she was running as a sprinter in junior athletics competitions. She won medals in national events and at a regional competition in Taipei. By June 2014, she had come to the attention of Indian sports authorities as a woman who may fall under the Sport Authority of India's (SAI) hyperandrogenism policy. Her medical evaluators concluded that she should not be permitted to compete in women's events until her androgen level was reduced to an "appropriate range." Dr. Payoshi Mitra, whose LinkedIn profile describes her as a researcher and activist in gender and sports, soon became an advisor to Chand. By September, Chand had written to the Athletics Federation of India (AFI) protesting her ineligibility, declining to have her medical records forwarded to the IAAF, and requesting support for her appeal to the Court of Arbitration for Sport (CAS).[13] Although the SAI's hyperandrogenism policy operated somewhat differently from the IAAF policy, the latter was Chand's and her supporters' ultimate target.

CAS TAKES CHARGE

CAS, with its main headquarters in Lausanne, Switzerland, was founded in 1984 and has become the preferred body for dealing with disputes within sport. (CAS rulings have on occasion been challenged in national courts.)[14] Chand and her allies made their case before a three-person arbitration panel in March 2015. Chand is an extraordinarily sympathetic plaintiff. Born to a family of weavers, she discovered a talent for and love of running. Like many gifted young athletes, she dedicated herself to perfecting that talent; running became central to her identity as a young woman. Her letter to the Secretary General of the AFI included this plea: " . . . I am unable to understand why I am asked to fix my body in a certain way simply for participation as a woman. I was born a woman, reared up as a woman, I identify as a woman and I believe I should be allowed to compete with other women . . . "[15] Her letter also included two claims supplied by unnamed experts: first, that the policy's basis was "unscientific"; and, second, that if she was to undergo medical treatment, the "interventions are invasive, often irreversible, and will harm my health now and in the future."[15] The second claim was refuted by expert witnesses who treat women with DSDs. In most cases, they reported, taking oral contraceptives such as those used by countless women around the world can reduce high testosterone levels.

Very little public information is available about what happens to hyperandrogenic women athletes. One scientific report describes four such women who underwent surgery. Chand's supporters suggested those women might have been pressured into agreeing to surgery thinking this would improve their chances of returning to competition. It's also possible they believed that surgery would improve their health and life. Those motives are not mutually exclusive, of course. (XY women have testes; those organs can become cancerous. Offering women the option of having them removed is a part of standard medical management in such cases.) All of the women were from rural or mountainous areas of developing countries. At least three, possibly all four, were biologically related. Athletes identified in the hyperandrogenism protocol get access to world-class experts for their medical management, and the IAAF protocol unequivocally does not *require* surgery for eligibility to be restored. Nonetheless, it's possible they felt intimidated by the professionals who recommended surgery.[16]

In its decision, the CAS panel rejected most of Chand's arguments, but it found grounds to allow her to continue to compete without having to be subject to the hyperandrogenism protocol— at least for two years.[15] Digging into the panel's conclusions and reasoning highlights some of the enduring challenges encountered at the intersection between the science of gender and the values of sport.

The CAS panel's judgment rested on two pillars: the right of every individual to participate in sport along with the IAAF experts' inability to prove conclusively that male levels of testosterone produced within a woman's own body confer a *significant* athletic advantage.

THE ANDROGEN ADVANTAGE

No one disputes that pills, patches, or injections of testosterone or its chemical knockoffs—synthetic anabolic steroids— significantly enhance performance. East Germany proved that beyond all doubt through its systematic doping of women athletes. But how great an advantage do women get who produce their own abundant testosterone? Is it in the one percent range? Or is it closer to the edge elite male athletes typically have over elite women competing in the same event? No number is universally accepted here, but the panel cited a range of 10–12 percent advantage for men with one of the expert's calculations closer to 13 percent. If women with hyperandrogenism derived a one percent advantage, that doesn't seem like much—at best a tenth of the typical male advantage, well within the range of other biological variations among elite athletes. If that's all the edge provided, there may be no need for a policy on hyperandrogenism that singles out certain women for their naturally occurring boost from testosterone. One of the experts, Dr. Stéphane Bermon, suggested three percent as a plausible estimate, though he also cautioned that no definitive scientific evidence is available. Three percent would amount to roughly a 3.5-second advantage in the women's 800-meter finals at the Rio Olympics, enough to make the difference between first and seventh place. The women finishing behind the runner(s) with a three-percent advantage might understandably regard that as significant.

If women with hyperandrogenism are indeed getting a substantial boost from their higher androgen levels, what should we do? Critics of the policy, so far at least, have said they accept that there should be separate competitions for women and for men. Advocates for women's participation in sport would be in an odd position if they argued otherwise.

Chand's advocates raise an important philosophical question: Should the relatively rare occurrence of hyperandrogenism in women be regarded as just another variation in natural talents, like the size of her hands, the length of her femur, her height, or her capacity to utilize oxygen? In a representative article, advocates argue that " . . . athletes never begin on a fair playing field; if they were not exceptional in one regard or another, they would not have made it to a prestigious international athletic stage."[17]

I believe the advocates make two mistakes here. First they dismiss the very idea of a fair playing field because, they say, exceptionally talented athletes have advantages over the less talented, and therefore not everyone has an equal chance to win. But the whole point of trying to create a fair and level playing field is precisely so talent (and dedication) can prevail. Is it fair to make 14-year-old cyclists race against 25-year-olds even though the younger cyclists will always lose? To insist that 120-pound wrestlers grapple with superheavyweights? To make women run against men? None of these scenarios is unfair, strictly speaking. As I've argued, though, fairness comes into play only after we've come to an understanding about meaning and values in the sport.

The second mistake, then, is the failure to ask whether the contest between women with and without a hyperandrogen advantage can be meaningful and interesting. Every sport that creates eligibility categories—whether by age, weight, or type and severity of impairment—has answered that question by staging separate events so that raw biological differences don't overwhelm talent, dedication, and courage. And with very few exceptions, every sport offers separate competitions for women and for men. Having competitions limited only to hyperandrogenic women isn't a realistic option. So, what can we do?

We should begin by acknowledging that no policy can be perfect. Whatever is decided, some people will be disadvantaged; some important values will fail to be fully honored. The attempt to impose rules and structure on the effervescent chaos of human biology and social organization inevitably leaves some people on the wrong side of the line. But that's no excuse for a poor policy.

POLICY OPTIONS

Perhaps nature will be kind. Perhaps so few women are born with a man's level of testosterone, strength, and power that women's sport can shrug off their impact the way Nordic skiing did with Eero Mäntyranta's genetically derived extra red blood cells. Mäntyranta, after all, lost far more races than he won.

Probably the simplest policy is to decree that every person who identifies as a woman has the right to participate in women's events. Some of the witnesses testifying on behalf of Chand suggested this option. It may be that such women are rare and would dominate very few competitions. If so, we might conclude that the frustration suffered by the women competing against them was outweighed by the loss of privacy or other possible harms to women athletes singled out for their male-like advantages. Others, of course, might strike the balance differently out of concern for the women who did not have the same advantages. In effect, by dividing a sport into women's and men's competitions we are declaring that being a man rather than a woman should *not* count as a relevant "natural talent" any more than being twenty-five rather than twelve years old.

The "simple" option turns out to be not quite so simple. We could take an individual's personal declaration that she is a woman as the final word. This has the merit of respecting the athlete's choice and privacy. Or we could require some sort of official document, perhaps a passport or driver's license attesting that the person is a woman. At least six countries now provide a gender option other than male or female. At this writing, four countries permit a person to choose their legal gender without any requirement for medical treatment or certification by a doctor.[18] More jurisdictions likely will follow as the rights of individuals who do not fit comfortably into the binary classifications of male and female are increasingly recognized. In late 2015, the IOC issued a new policy on eligibility for transgender athletes. Individuals who transition from female to male may compete without restriction. Those transitioning from male to female, on the other hand, must maintain a testosterone level below 10 nmol/L—the same standard proposed in the hyperandrogenism policy.[19] The challenge faced by sport is how to accommodate victories for gender-related human rights into competitions that, until now, relied on precisely that binary division in order to give women a chance to succeed.

Unfortunately, the possibility of abuse cannot be ignored. The same dynamic that drives athletes to use performance-enhancing drugs may result in some presenting themselves as women, including XY males. If you're talented, but not quite talented enough to beat other men, the option of competing against women may look attractive. If you live in a country where all you have to do to become a woman by law is to say so, and if sport agrees to recognize as a woman anyone who can produce an attesting document, perhaps social pressure or shaming would discourage such behavior. The person would likely have to live as a woman, which is fine if your gender identity coincides with your "sport" gender. But shaming and questioning an athlete's gender is ugly and demeaning—certainly not much gain of moral ground.

And the abuse won't always be the individual athlete's idea. The athlete's ecosystem—coaches, trainers, team officials, sponsors, even national sports authorities—have much to gain by an athlete's success. Just as some of these mini-ecosystems pushed athletes to dope, we can expect some to look for ways to exploit whatever cracks appear in sport's eligibility rules. A plausible, though by no means certain, consequence of a policy that accepts an individual's self-declaration of gender will be to disadvantage women who don't have the physical advantages of men.

The Federation of Gay Games organizes competitions that acknowledge the complexity and fluidity of gender. At the same time, it recognizes that men typically have athletic advantages, and it wants to give women the chance to succeed by competing against other women. Therefore, the Federation's policy guidelines on "Gender in Sport" require that "certain competition categories must be reserved for women."[20] Organizers also can have a men's division, a mixed division, or both. The Federation accepts typical legal documents as proof of gender, but it also acknowledges that "legal and medical systems of various countries, and the individual situations of participants, may make the use of legal gender insufficient or inappropriate for the purposes of defining whether a participant competes as a male or female." The Federation's gender classification policy unfortunately can't escape the quandaries of the simple solution. It still has to decide who is eligible to compete as a woman. The concept of a mixed division is intriguing and could gain traction beyond the Gay Games. In any case, here we see an organization wholeheartedly committed both to sport and to full recognition of gender and sexual diversity struggling with many of the same questions that puzzle other sports governing bodies.

We cannot know how the CAS panel might have ruled if Dutee Chand had been allowed to compete in a mixed division. Her human right to participate in sport would have been recognized. But as long as people remain ignorant of the diversity of human sexuality and gender, and until persons who don't fit neatly into the male-female binary can embrace this knowledge without feeling shame, sport will struggle to balance respect for difference with fairness. There is absolutely no question that people such as Semenya and Chand must be treated with respect and their dignity as persons recognized unconditionally. At the same time, women should be allowed to have fair and meaningful competitions. There is much work left to do on the science of hyperandrogenism and athletic performance, and a great deal of hard thinking ahead on the best policy for deciding who is eligible to compete in women's events. We should start by focusing on the meanings and values in sport. That may not give us a rapid or simple answer, but it will assure that we're asking the right questions.

Although dramatic changes in social attitudes toward sex and gender can be agonizingly slow, change is possible. In a remarkably short time, the right of gay persons to marry in the United States and in other nations has gone from nearly unthinkable to how-could-we-possibly-have-thought-otherwise? (To be sure, the groundwork for changing public opinion and public policy was many years in the making.) Whatever else we do now, we can support the work of people trying to dispel ignorance and assure the rights of persons who don't fit neatly into the binary. The closer we approach that goal, the less stigma and shame anyone would have to endure.

Just in case you might have hoped a simple solution would resolve the quandary, consider what has happened with Semenya since CAS's decision in the Chand case. After returning to competition in 2010, Semenya had a respectable competitive career. Since the IAAF's hyperandrogenism policy was suspended, however, she has become dominant. In the April 2016 South African championships, Semenya beat her personal best in the 400 meters by nearly two seconds, ran a world's best time of the year in the 800 meters, and for good measure also easily won the 1500-meter race. Ross Tucker, a prominent South African sports scientist noted: "She looks ridiculously lean and athletic. She's a different athlete compared with last year."[21] Speculation has begun that, with the IAAF's policy set aside, she was no longer required to take testosterone-suppressing medications in order to remain eligible to compete as a woman. Semenya won gold in the 800 meters in the 2016 Summer Olympics with a time of 1:55.28, better than her performance in Berlin in 2009 and good for eleventh place on the all-time list for the women's 800 meters. It should be noted that many of the performances ranking ahead of her occurred during an era when doping was rampant. No one is accusing Semenya of doping. But it's noteworthy that so many of those other record-setting performances by women were possible only with the aid of androgenic hormones. If, indeed, Semenya's body makes abundant testosterone, she also is getting an androgenic boost that her non-hyperandrogenic competitors are not. Some of the women who raced against her in the final heat in Rio seemed not to see it as a fair and meaningful contest.[22] Doing justice to all concerned will not be easy or comfortable but everyone committed to fairness in women's sport must make the effort.

NOTES

1. Smith D. Report claims 800m world champion Caster Semenya is a hermaphrodite. *The Guardian* [Internet]. 2009 Sep 10 [cited 2016 Jul 28]. Available from: https://www.theguardian.com/sport/2009/sep/10/caster-semenya-hermaphrodite-iaaf-test.
2. Callow J. Caster Semenya faces growing backlash after competitors have their say. *The Guardian* [Internet]. 2010 Aug 23 [cited 2016 Jul 28]. Available from: https://www.theguardian.com/sport/2010/aug/23/caster-semenya-backlash-jemma-simpson.
3. Govender P. South African Semenya cleared to return. *Reuters* [Internet]. 2010 Jul 6 [cited 2016 Jul 28]. Available from: http://www.reuters.com/article/us-athletics-semenya-idUSTRE6652M320100706.
4. Carlson A. When is a woman not a woman? For 24 years Maria Patino thought she was female. Then she failed the sex test? *Womens Sport Fit.* 1991 Mar;24–29.
5. Martínez-Patiño MJ. Personal account: A woman tried and tested. Special Issue: Medicine and Sport. *The Lancet.* 2005;9503:S38.
6. Martínez-Patiño MJ. Maria Jose Martinez Patiño Personal Communication. 2016.
7. Berg S. 1936 Berlin Olympics: How Dora the man competed in the woman's high Jump [Internet]. *Der Spiegel Online.* 2009 Sept 15 [cited 2016 Feb 9]. Available from: http://www.spiegel.de/international/germany/1936-berlin-olympics-how-dora-the-man-competed-in-the-woman-s-high-jump-a-649104.html.

8. Sakamoto H, Nakanoin K, Komatsu H, Michimoto T, Takashima E, Furuyama J. Femininity control at the XXth Universiade in Kobe, Japan. *Int J Sports Med.* 1988;9(3):193–195.

9. Reeser JC. Gender identity and sport: Is the playing field level? *Br J Sports Med.* 2005 Oct;39(10):695–699.

10. Elsas LJ, Ljungqvist A, Ferguson-Smith MA, Simpson JL, Genel M, Carlson A, et al. Gender verification of female athletes. *Genetic Med.* 2000;2(4):249–254.

11. Genel M, Ljungqvist A. Gender verification of female athletes. *Lancet.* 2005 Dec;366(Medicine and Sport):S41.

12. Bermon S, Garnier PY, Lindén Hirschberg A, Robinson N, Giraud S, Nicoli R, et al. Serum androgen levels in elite female athletes. *J Clin Endocrinol Metab.* 2014 Nov;99(11):4328–4335.

13. Sengupta R. Why Dutee Chand can change sports [Internet]. *Live Mint.* 2014 Nov 24 [cited 2016 Feb 12]. Available from: http://www.livemint. com/Leisure/9P3jbOG2G0ppTVB7Xvwj0K/Why-Dutee-Chand-can-change-sports.html.

14. Coletta A. Speedskater is poised to upend rule of sports' highest court. *New York Times* [Internet]. 2016 Feb 11 [cited 2016 Feb 12]. Available from: http://www.nytimes.com/2016/02/12/sports/skater-challenges-supremacy-of-court-of-arbitration-for-sport.html.

15. Court of Arbitration for Sport. *Interim Arbitral Award Dutee Chand v. AFI & IAAF* [Internet]. (2015). Available from: http://www.tas-cas. org/fileadmin/user_upload/award_internet.pdf.

16. Fénichel P, Paris F, Philibert P, Hiéronimus S, Gaspari L, Kurzenne J-Y, et al. Molecular diagnosis of 5α-reductase deficiency in 4 elite young female athletes through hormonal screening for hyperandrogenism. *J Clin Endocrinol Metab.* 2013 Jun;98(6):E1055–E1059.

17. Karkazis K, Jordan-Young R, Davis G, Camporesi S. Out of bounds? A critique of the new policies on hyperandrogenism in elite female athletes. *Am J Bioeth.* 2012 Jul;12(7):3–16.

18. McDonald H. Ireland passes law allowing trans people to choose their legal gender. *The Guardian* [Internet]. 2015 Jul 16 [cited 2016 Feb 12]. Available from: http://www.theguardian.com/world/2015/jul/16/ireland-transgender-law-gender-recognition-bill-passed.

19. IOC. IOC consensus meeting on sex reassignment and hyperandrogenism. Nov 2015 [Internet]. [cited 2017 Jan 2]. Available from: http://www. triathlon.org/uploads/docs/6.b_2015.11_IOC_consensus_meeting_on_ sex_reassignment_and_hyperandrogenism-ENG.pdf.

20. Federation of Gay Games. Gender in sport [Internet]. 2017. Available from: https://gaygames.org/wp/sport/sports-policiesd/gender/

21. Ingle S. British athletes demand stronger action from WADA on drug cheats. *The Guardian* [Internet]. 2016 Jun 13 [cited 2016 Jun 22].

Available from: https://www.theguardian.com/sport/2016/jun/13/ british-athletes-letter-world-anti-doping-agency-drug-cheats.

22. Bull A. Caster Semenya wins gold but faces more scrutiny as IAAF press case. *The Guardian* [Internet]. 2016 Aug 21 [cited 2016 Aug 26]. Available from: https://www.theguardian.com/sport/2016/aug/21/ caster-semenya-wins-gold-but-faces-scrutiny.

Chapter 7

Using—and Misusing—
Health and Safety

I can't see any ethical difference between giving a drug to improve performance and wrapping an ankle or handing out a salt pill for the same purpose. Athletes hear about these things, and they are going to get them one way or another.

Dr. H. Kay Dooling

The ethical paradox of elite sports medicine is that a physician can collaborate in harming the patient by accepting his "right" to be treated as he wishes.

John Hoberman

In 1998, Juan Antonio Samaranch, then President of the International Olympic Committee, said, "Doping [now] is everything that, firstly, is harmful to an athlete's health and, secondly, artificially augments his performance. If it's just the second case, for me that's not doping. If it's the first case, it is."[1] With that declaration, Samaranch made his contribution to the unfortunate tradition of ill-conceived pronouncements about athletes and performance-enhancing drugs.

When I began my investigations into the ethics of performance-enhancing drugs, the "experts" were convinced there were two reasons to keep them out of sport: They made competitions unfair, and they imperiled athletes' health. The concern for fairness, I've argued, is better understood as the desire to preserve meanings and values in sport. Both supporters and critics of anti-doping, meanwhile, have wielded health as an argument for their stance.

There were plausible reasons to worry about the well-being of doping athletes in 1980. The drugs of choice were anabolic steroids and amphetamines. There were credible reports of professional football players coming down hard after taking loads of stimulants before games, cereal bowls full of "uppers" in Major League Baseball clubhouses, and athletes taking massive doses of steroids far beyond the recommended therapeutic amounts.[2]

The evidence regarding doping's impact on health at the time was anecdotal. There's a wise saying in science: "The plural of anecdote is not data." Dramatic stories are one thing, reliable data quite another. Solid scientific evidence on the health impacts of PEDs was scarce. Few scientists were interested; funding was almost nonexistent; and athletes were loath to admit they were using PEDs, let alone to cooperate with investigators. Research ethics was a further obstacle. In response to revelations about the mistreatment of human research subjects, the National Commission for the Protection of Human Subjects of Biomedical and Behavioral Research was created in the 1970s. The Commission offered guidance on specific topics, including research on prisoners and on children. It also advocated for independent ethical review of proposals that would use human subjects.

Put yourself in the place of a researcher who somehow had the interest and the support to conduct a well-designed study that would give huge doses of powerful drugs to healthy young people—not to treat disease, mind you, just to see what impact the drugs had on their sports performance and their health. The review committees, known as IRBs, short for "institutional review boards," might have been dumbfounded. You want to do *what*? Expose people to possibly catastrophic risks, with no medical benefit to anyone? In the decades following, athletes and scientists found clever ways to extract useful information without violating research ethics rules. But even now, there are disagreements over the impact on health for many PEDs.[3]

Anti-doping skeptics argue that the risks are exaggerated and that athletes' health would be better served by permitting doping. One influential article offered this proposal: "An alternative policy might involve making legal the use of drugs associated with low harm and testing health rather than testing for drugs. Implicit in this argument is that more athletes would use performance-enhancing drugs if they were both legal and safe, thereby obviating both the moral and level playing field problems. This view holds that if health is safeguarded it does not matter how performance is supplemented."[4] (p87) Samaranch would agree with the last sentence.

If this suggestion were adopted more athletes would use drugs, of course. And not only elite athletes; more on that later. The competitive dynamic that drive athletes to use PEDs in the first place makes it highly unlikely that they will use only the "safe" drugs, and only in the doses and combinations recommended by their medical advisors. The proposal also will encounter practical difficulties. What criteria will be used to decide which drugs and dosages are safe? Who will be entrusted with that judgment? The US Food and Drug Administration and its counterpart, the European Medicines Agency, are unlikely to embrace anything remotely like this charge. Judgments about safety also can change as we learn more about risks. EPO, for example, was widely regarded as a safe drug for boosting the number of red blood cells—until evidence mounted that it was killing some of the people taking it to treat anemia. These patients were generally aiming for a modest boost—just enough to give them a bit more energy—not the physiological extremes sought by cyclists and other athletes.

In 2004, Savulescu and colleagues proposed prohibiting anabolic steroids but allowing EPO. They wrote: "Taking EPO up to the safe level, say 0.5, is not a problem. This allows athletes to correct for natural inequality. There are of course some drugs that are harmful in themselves—for example, anabolic steroids. We should focus on detecting these because they are harmful not because they enhance performance."[5] [(p668)]

The number they gave, 0.5, is for red cells as a proportion of whole blood. The FDA calibrates its recommendations to the level of hemoglobin rather than packed cell volume, or hematocrit, as it's also known. The 0.5 concentration deemed harmless by Savulescu translates to a hemoglobin of 16.7. In its 24 June 2011 announcement, the FDA cited three large-scale studies of patients with kidney failure who were treated with ESAs—erythropoiesis stimulating agents—that is, EPO and its variants. The FDA press release was blunt: The use of ESAs increases the risk of cardiovascular events such as stroke, thrombosis, and death.[6] There was also evidence that ESAs can cause tumors to grow. One of the studies found the risk of stroke nearly doubled in the people who took ESAs—and that was with a median hemoglobin level of 12.5—far below the 16.7 touted as "safe" by Savulescu. ESAs have been required to carry a "black box" warning since 2007 about the dangers accompanying their use, a warning known to pharmaceutical marketers as the "kiss of death."

Not all of this evidence was available when Savulescu and his colleagues argued that athletes should be permitted to use EPO. And the people in these studies are older and sicker than the athletes likely to use it, so the risks may be less dire in healthy young people. But the claim that EPO is entirely benign is naive at best.

No one can assure fit young athletes who push their hematocrits to fifty percent and beyond that they aren't risking their health. The reports of European cyclists dropping dead shortly after EPO first hit the market may have served as a bizarre sort of reassurance for other bike racers: "We're not hearing reports of cyclists dropping like flies anymore, so EPO must be safe as long as you don't massively overdose." Nevertheless, evidence shows that ESAs can cause serious health problems, and young cyclists cannot be confident that they're somehow exempt.

The EPO story serves as a more general caution for anyone hoping to offer a list of "safe" drugs that athletes can use with impunity. We can justify accepting risks that come with potent drugs in order to treat a serious illness. The risk calculation is different with healthy young athletes. They may be all too willing to jeopardize their health tomorrow if they believe the drugs will help them win today. Furthermore, using PEDs may not have been their idea in the first place; people who benefit from their athletic success may have prodded them into using drugs.

An intriguing feature of Kayser and Smith's proposal is the idea of testing for "health" rather than the presence of drugs. Just what would physicians look for as measures of health? Athletes' physiology can diverge widely from the norms established in healthy people. What indices will be used to decide that an athlete has crossed the line from healthy to unhealthy? That's one problem. A larger challenge is figuring out how to gauge long-term risks to health. Will we be able to detect early warning signs? Or will those early signals, if they appear at all, be lost in the physiological noise of young bodies stressed by intense training? Until we have a better grasp of what it would mean to test for health in young athletes using drugs in the quest for enhanced performance, the eagerness to embrace widespread use of PEDs seems hasty.

Recent attacks against anti-doping often take a "let's keep throwing mud on the wall and see what sticks" approach. Charges leveled against the effort to keep performance-enhancing drugs out of sport include that it's misguided, unfair, confused, and wasteful; that it violates athletes' privacy; and that it drives drug use underground. Skeptics toss additional arguments such as: A ban may nudge athletes to use drugs that are more difficult to detect, even if those drugs might be more dangerous than the alternatives; prohibited drugs are likely to come from unregulated black market suppliers with all the risks of contamination and inaccurate dosages typical of that world; and athletes may be less willing to be honest with their doctors about what they're using, compromising their physicians' ability to provide optimal care. This last observation buttresses proposals to put doping under physicians' control. Unfortunately, there are reasons to worry that this strategy may not be as promising as it sounds.

THE HARM-REDUCTION STRATEGY

Physician involvement in doping has a long history. Proposals to put doctors openly and officially in control rely on a strategy that has had success with conventional drug abuse. Heroin addicts and others have been helped through "harm reduction" programs. Injection drug users can be provided clean needles rather than sharing possibly contaminated needles with other users to avoid spreading infections such as HIV. The drugs they inject can come from a trustworthy agency rather than from unreliable black-market suppliers. They're still using the drugs, and individuals are still risking their health, but the overall health of the population of drug users is not as bad as it would have been had these programs not existed. Thus the strategy's name: Harm *reduction*.

Medical supervision and harm reduction for performance-enhancing drug use in athletes has advantages in theory over the current policy of prohibition. We could learn more about which drugs were dangerous if athletes used them openly and scientists could more easily study their impact. Athletes would have no reason to choose hard-to-detect drugs that might be more dangerous than their more easily detectable alternatives. And athletes would no longer face the dangers of contamination and mislabeling that come with black-market sources.

Proponents of harm reduction as a response to PEDs in sport concede that their use likely would rise as a consequence. Unfortunately, our experience with the dynamic driving PED use in sport doesn't inspire faith that athletes would limit themselves to the drugs and dosages prescribed by their doctors.

The analogy with the harm-reduction strategy for drugs of abuse such as heroin quickly falls apart. Heroin users don't compete with each other to see who can get highest. They want enough of the drug to satisfy their craving. Athletes, on the other hand, want to get higher—or faster, or stronger, to borrow from the Olympic motto—than any other athlete. When it comes to using performance-enhancing drugs, the goal is to do more or better than everyone else.

The comforting vision of athletes going to their physicians for benign doses of drugs that science has proved are safe to use is not grounded in reality. If a "harm-reduction" strategy were introduced into sport, athletes would get drugs that enhance performance from their doctors. In fact, any athlete who hopes to remain in contention will feel compelled to take whatever drugs are permitted because everyone they're lining up against is under the same pressure to use the approved drugs rather than surrender any advantage to their competitors. Drug use won't just rise a little. In every sport where drugs are believed to make a difference, use will become more or less compulsory. Competing without PEDs would be like a modern tennis player using a wooden racket: He or she might consider this a more "pure" expression of the sport, but such a choice would undermine any chance at competitive success.

Athletes who refuse PEDs will find themselves at the back of the pack, or they'll just give up competing. Some exceptions will remain: the Edwin Moseses of the world whose superior talents and dedication allow them to compete successfully without drugs. But such exceptions will prove the rule. Merely mortal athletes will face the three regrettable choices I described in chapter 1. They can decline to use PEDs, knowing their competitors are using and will probably prevail; drop down or out of that level of competition; or try to match whatever doping they believe the competition is doing.

Under a "harm reduction" policy for PEDs in sport, the "officially approved" drugs will become the mandatory floor. The relentless quest for competitive advantage will drive athletes to try larger dosages of the permitted drugs. Some will pile other, unapproved drugs on top of the ones their physician provides. In the end, athletes will take drugs in combinations and dosages for which no one understands the risks. The forces that drive today's PED use aren't going away. We know that athletes will blow past the permitted limits. It's hard to see how this could be good for athletes' health. Any responsible physician who understands the dynamics of PED use in competitive sport would have to pause before endorsing—or participating—in the medicalization of doping. And unless "testing for health," including long-term health, turns out to be far easier and more reliable than seems plausible, anti-doping will have to continue much as it does today. Harm reduction is an appealing option in theory. But where heroin users want enough to satisfy their craving, athletes want more than the other guy, and that makes all the difference.

PHYSICIAN INVOLVEMENT IN DOPING: THE DARK SIDE

The history of physician involvement with doping reinforces our concerns. Robert Kerr, a California physician, boasted of writing thousands of prescriptions for anabolic steroids for athletes, bodybuilders, and cops. By 1986 he claimed to have stopped providing steroids to athletes: They wouldn't use them as prescribed. In a 1990 interview, he said "The athletes duped me . . . If two drugs are good, they're going to 'stack' those two with three or 10 or 15. I do not think it is the right thing for doctors to get involved in the steroid business."[7 (p1699)]

A sobering study of physicians' involvement with sports doping by John Hoberman reveals that physicians can be very creative at excusing what they do with the athletes in their "care." He reports that five of the leading sports physicians in West Germany in 1976 publicly endorsed medically supervised administration of steroids to athletes. Fifteen years later, another West German sports physician noted that dealing with elite athletes sometimes required decisions weighing health against performance. "An important factor is the courage required of the doctor to really engage the patient's condition, and there are only a few practitioners who are capable of that," he proclaimed. There is something fundamentally creepy about a doctor describing himself as "courageous" because he is abetting cheating by athletes, jeopardizing his patients' health, and collaborating in a scheme that pushes other athletes to take similar risks. Hoberman wryly notes: "The ethical paradox of elite sports medicine is that a physician can collaborate in harming the patient by accepting his 'right' to be treated as he wishes."[8] [(p207)] Ivan Waddington points out the disconnect between the image of sports medicine as the "front line" in the battle against doping versus the reality that sports physicians have been important developers and disseminators of PEDs.[9]

A physician working at a US Olympic training camp in 1968 defended medically supervised steroids for athletes. The arguments he offered anticipated more recent attacks on anti-doping. Dr. H. Kay Dooling told an interviewer for *Sports Illustrated*: "I don't pretend to be a researcher or a scientist, I'm a practicing physician who is interested in athletes. A lot of physicians are stuffed shirts when it comes to sports. Athletes do want to perform better, that is what it is all about. If I know of something which may improve performance, a training or rehabilitation technique, a drug that is legal and which I don't believe involves any serious health risk, I see no reason not to make it available to an athlete. I can't see any ethical difference between giving a drug to improve performance and wrapping an ankle or handing out a salt pill for the same purpose. Athletes hear about these things and they are going to get them one way or another."[10] [(p5)]

Dr. Dooling packs a number of common but dubious assumptions into that statement. First, that all methods of enhancing performance are ethically indistinguishable. This echoes the argument that seeks to obliterate all distinctions among the multitude of ways athletes can improve their performances: wraps are like salt pills are like anabolic steroids are like better equipment and so on. Second, because athletes will find a way to get whatever they want, I, their physician, am morally blameless if they get it from me instead of some clandestine lab. And third, the only good reason to deny them a drug is my belief that it's a risk to their health.

The claim that all distinctions are incoherent when it comes to improving sports performance doesn't survive even a modest poke. Sport creates meaning in part by the limits it sets on the means of enhancing performance. Someone could cover the 26.2 miles of a marathon on roller skates faster than any runner, but they wouldn't deserve to win, even if the organizers had failed to prohibit using wheels. (Rosie Ruiz used a different set of wheels in the 1979 New York City marathon: She took the subway on her way to the finish line of that city's race. Six months later, her apparent victory in the Boston marathon was overturned when witnesses reported they'd seen her emerge from a crowd of bystanders near the finish.) The issue is not whether to draw lines—we have to do that or else gut the meaning of sport—but where we draw them and what principles we rely on to do so.

Dooling's second assumption concerns physicians' ethical obligations to their patients. Patients may request a drug that the doctor sincerely believes would do them no good. But perhaps it would do no harm either, and patients might take prescribing it as a sign that the doctor really cared for them. Placebos can help people feel better at times. Dr. Dooling overlooks a fundamental distinction: Giving a drug under a harm-reduction program to a heroin addict affects mainly that patient; whatever knock-on effects it has are predominantly positive—for example, that person will not need to resort to crime to get his next fix. Physicians should know that providing performance-enhancing drugs to their patient affects not only that patient's health; it also puts malign pressures on other athletes—and their doctors—to do the same.

Finally, Dr. Dooling proudly admits he is not a researcher or scientist. Yet he seems quite willing to rely on his own belief that the drugs he's handing out are not harmful. When the evidence that the drug is harmless—short- and long-term—is scant or nonexistent, as it was in 1969 for steroids, and remains today for many drugs sought by athletes, how is a responsible physician supposed to weigh the risks and advise his or her patients? Especially when the purpose of the drug is not to cure disease, relieve symptoms, or prevent injury, but to boost performance? It's one thing to rely on therapeutic judgment in the absence of solid science when treating serious medical problems, quite another to tinker with the bodies of healthy young persons merely to boost their athletic performance.

The picture would be incomplete without noting that physicians who cater to athletes seeking banned PEDs are also furthering their own interests. Doctors derive income and status from their connection with elite athletes. Hoberman notes that " . . . doctors are frequently tempted to deemphasize the athlete's status as a patient in favor of treating him or her as a commercially valuable asset whose performances take precedence over genuine medical needs."[11] (p250)

Because sports doping is driven by a fundamentally different dynamic than heroin abuse, and because physicians cannot always be counted on to look first after an athlete's health, we'd be foolish to rely on medically supervised doping to reduce harm. Nor, it turns out, does it avoid all those chunks of mud clinging to the wall. If, inevitably, some athletes will want to use more and different drugs than doctors prescribe, how will we assure the athletes who want to play within the new rules that they're not once again on a tilted field? We'll need some way to identify athletes who go beyond what's allowed.

In other words, we'll need a system of testing and sanctions that may look a lot like our current anti-doping system. All the moaning about invasions of privacy, inconvenience, expense, unfairness, and the like is beside the point. Some version of the current apparatus of doping control may be as indispensable to a system of medically supervised doping as it is to one that bans doping altogether.

Unless we are willing to allow athletes to use anything and everything—that is, physicians supervising unlimited drug use—and unless there is an extraordinarily happy circumstance such that the typical doctor following the typical athlete will be able to know every time that athlete veers from the prescribed path, then we'll just be moving the goalposts. Drawing a line between good and bad drugs and dosages won't clear the mud from the wall. But it will mean near universal drug use in sports where PEDs are effective. And not merely for elite athletes. Not for only adult athletes, either. Young people who want to emulate their heroes will want to know which drugs they're relying on to boost performance. Once doping is rendered a normal, accepted, endorsed practice, the consequences are likely to be far reaching.

DOPING, CONTAGION, AND PUBLIC HEALTH

However concerned we are about the health effects of high-dose multiple drug use among elite adult athletes, the likely impact on younger athletes is vastly more worrisome. And the numbers are huge.

More than two million American boys and girls participate in Little League. USA Baseball estimates that more than five million Americans of all ages play baseball—and that leaves out the many who play in Parks and Recreation Leagues. The numbers of Americans playing soccer are astounding. FIFA's 2006 Big Count estimated that twenty-four million play soccer in the United States, including four million in registered youth programs. The largest such program, US Youth Soccer, has more than three million enrolled participants, an increase of 90 percent since the 1990–1991 season. The United States' 4.3 million registered soccer competitors (a number that includes adults) is second only to Germany's 6.3 million, and more than twice that of Brazil. For female soccer players, the United States has twice as many registered players as any other nation.

Football is by far the most popular sport among American high school boys with over 1.1 million participants in 2015–2016 (the most recent period in the statistics compiled by the National Federation of State High School Associations.) Track and field (indoor plus outdoor) has roughly equal numbers of girls and boys, over 1.2 million participants in total. Nearly a million high school students played basketball. Baseball and softball together add up to over 860,000 with soccer next at roughly 820,000 team participants.[12]

Young amateurs are far less likely than elite adult athletes to have access to sports medicine specialists. Their coaches have less experience spotting or dealing with players using performance-enhancing drugs. And many of the drugs athletes use, including powerful hormones such as anabolic steroids, have more profound effects at earlier stages of human development.

If performance-enhancing drugs become openly and widely used by elite athletes, accepted by sport, and seen as a necessary ingredient for athletic success, the message will be resoundingly clear to college and high school athletes, echoing down through the ranks of the youngest would-be competitors. What will youth sport be like when wanting to "be like Mike" means not just having enormous talent, incredible discipline, and an insatiable desire to excel, but also taking a bit of hGH, a course of EPO, some anabolic steroids, and an amphetamine top-up at game time? Body builders and power lifters already endorse products that claim to build muscle mass, definition, and strength. It's a small stretch to imagine famous basketball, football, and baseball players signing up to promote some company's version of EPO, testosterone, or whatever other drugs can be peddled to credulous teens.

Limiting performance-enhancing drug use to elite athletes carefully supervised by expert clinicians is an improbable fantasy. Young aspiring athletes will want access to the same drugs as their role models. They'll get them through their not-so-expert physician or, if their doctor won't cooperate, from other sources not as scrupulous or accountable. The history of drug use in sport warns us that at least some coaches, trainers, and others who benefit when their athletes succeed won't object; in fact, they may prod their athletes to use drugs. Sadly, this may be true not only of elite and professional sports, but of college, high school, and youth leagues in which competitive success can advance the coach's career.

The likely outcome? A rolling public health epidemic.

HEALTH, DOPING, AND HEALING

When doping threatens athletes' health, preventing harm is a cogent reason to discourage it. Of course, there are plenty of things dangerous to athletes' health that have nothing to do with drugs—rules that encourage them to take extreme risks, for example. Women's gymnastics permits a vault known as the Produnova, after the first gymnast to land it successfully. It requires two and a half flips in the air. Aimee Boorman, noted Olympic gymnastics coach, said of the Produnova, "You land too far, you break your leg . . . You land too short, you break your neck. Or you die."[13]

There's a common argument in Bioethics: If something we prohibit is not notably worse than other things we allow, we should permit the banned thing as well. Savulescu employs this strategy when he writes in favor of permitting a drug only recently banned: " . . . meldonium, if clearly and accurately dosed, is unlikely to be more dangerous than many practices that we accept: training and full contact, or other permitted substances, such as caffeine."[14] [(p301)] This argument misunderstands the role health risks play in the ethics of performance-enhancing drugs in sport.

The simple fact that something adds a risk to someone's health is neither necessary nor sufficient to justify banning it. Of all the drugs that plagued bike racing, EPO was the most powerful. It increased endurance dramatically. A cyclist not using EPO would have no chance to win against others with talents roughly equal, or even slightly inferior, if they were injecting it. The same was true for cross-country ski racers. Imagine, though, that ski patrol workers discovered that EPO boosted their ability to rescue lost or injured skiers and return safely home. No one would object that they'd "artificially" enhanced their performance. After all, the purpose of ski rescue is to save lives without losing your own. If EPO contributed to that goal, terrific! The remaining ethical concern would be: Are they risking their own health unreasonably by using EPO?

Imagine another case. A neurosurgeon who specialized in the most delicate, risky operations is bothered by the slight hand tremors we all experience. She worries that those tremors interfere with her ability to perform precise operations on the most essential brain tissues. Our hypothetical neurosurgeon notices that a drug in common use, apparently quite safe, has as a side effect reducing tremors. She tries operating after taking the drug and believes her fine motor control is improved. Being a scientist at heart, she organizes a randomly assigned, placebo-controlled, double-blinded clinical trial with her colleagues. The result? Patients whose surgeons took the drug had fewer complications and swifter recoveries. The ethical question? How could you *not* use the drug when you operate? A surgeon who disdained the drug because it was an "artificial" enhancement should get the same response as one who insisted on using 19th-century surgical instruments on the grounds that they allowed him better to demonstrate his virtuosity. The point of surgery is to heal your patient. If taking a harmless drug contributes to your patients' recovery, use it. It's not about you; it's about the people in your care.

Performance-enhancing drugs in sport are an ethical problem in two ways: They undermine what's meaningful and valuable; and, given the pressure on athletes never to surrender a competitive advantage, permitting doping invites an avoidable public health disaster. Yet there may be circumstances where a flat-out prohibition is hard to justify.

Athletes get hurt. Even noncontact sports such as baseball see many injuries over the course of a season. Pitchers are particularly vulnerable to arm injuries. Throwing a baseball more than 90 miles per hour puts enormous stress on the elbow, especially on the ulnar collateral ligament, which connects two bones: the humerus in the upper arm to the ulna in the lower arm. In 1974, Tommy John, a successful pitcher, had a torn UCL replaced surgically with a tendon from another part of his body. After a rehabilitation lasting more than a year, he was able to return to the majors. Since then, the procedure now known as "Tommy John" surgery has been performed many times. Twenty-five percent of all pitchers in the Major Leagues had undergone the procedure according to the most recent authoritative survey. Although the numbers are small, fully 77 percent of active Major League baseball pitchers between 31 and 35 years old had had it.[15]

Tommy John surgery has helped thousands recover from a very serious injury. Unfortunately, there's a widespread belief that it enhances performance. This myth probably contributes to the disturbing number of young people who've had Tommy John surgery. Fifty-one percent of high school athletes believe that the surgery enhances pitchers' performances and should be performed on healthy arms.[16] The evidence is reasonably clear that it does not. After Tommy John surgery, pitchers typically lose speed off their fastball and give up more hits, walks, and earned runs—crucial measures of success—than before.[17] Some pitchers are able to throw faster after surgery and the long rehabilitation that follows. But experts attribute any increase in performance to the improved strength and conditioning achieved through rehab, not the surgery itself.

At times, athletes use banned drugs under morally ambiguous circumstances. Andy Pettitte, a very successful pitcher, admitted to injecting human growth hormone in what he claimed was an effort to speed healing of an injured pitching arm in 2002 and again in 2004. He denied ever using anabolic steroids. The scientific evidence for growth hormone as an aid to healing is scant; the FDA has not approved it for this purpose. But suppose there was solid evidence that a drug banned as a PED could significantly accelerate recovery from injury. If you weren't an elite athlete, your physician wouldn't hesitate to treat you with the drug. Is it reasonable to prohibit athletes from using a therapy available to nonathletes because it also might be used to gain a performance edge?

The examples of the ski rescuer and the innovative neurosurgeon demonstrate that drugs that enhance performance are not inherently problematic. Whether an athlete should be permitted to use an otherwise banned PED to recover from injury depends on the impact on meanings and values in sport along with any threat to health such use might pose. Baseball makes no exceptions for hGH even when athletes claim they're using it only to recover from injury. One reason offered is the lack of evidence that hGH aids recovery. If it did, and if that was the only benefit—if hGH did not result in lasting performance gains— then an athlete could take it while recuperating and stop using it long before resuming play, without any effect on post-recovery performance. Athletes could return to the field faster—a good thing—without enhancing their performance, the thing anti-doping tries to deter.

One line of argument blurs the distinction between routine training and serious injury. When you lift weights to build muscle, you cause microscopic damage to your tissues. During recovery from a workout, your body rebuilds those muscles to make them stronger than before. Healing from (microscopic, intentional) injury is an essential component of training. The training-as-injury-to-drugs-for-healing connection has been used to defend performance-enhancing substances such as steroids. After all, the argument goes, we're just trying to improve healing. Muscles will heal without steroids, of course, but without the extra anabolic kick steroids provide.

On the whole, though, healing from a serious injury seems different from normal training. For one thing, the damage wasn't voluntarily inflicted like the micro-injuries from training. For another, if we buy the idea that it's okay to use anabolic steroids to recover from the micro-injuries caused by intense training, the barn door is now wide open. This is exactly why and how athletes use anabolic steroids. On the whole, it makes sense to maintain the distinction between recovering from routine training and healing from serious injury.

The case for allowing injured athletes to use otherwise banned drugs while they heal seems strong. There is an avenue to permit this: the TUE, or therapeutic use exemption. TUEs also are used to try to be fair to athletes with long-term or chronic conditions who have a legitimate medical reason, and no good alternatives, for using an otherwise banned drug. There are also good reasons for sport to worry about athletes using purported injuries or illnesses to get access to PEDs. An incident from my time on the USOC's anti-doping committee stands out. A young man's cancerous testicles had to be removed. He could no longer produce a normal male level of testosterone. Standard medical treatment for a man who lost his testicles for medical reasons includes replacing what he lost with exogenous testosterone. He asked our committee for permission to receive testosterone therapy, monitored by a physician, to get his testosterone level back into the normal male range. I thought this was a reasonable request and was surprised to be in the minority. Finally, I asked my fellow committee members if they thought other athletes might have their testicles removed just so that they could take testosterone. (I may have used a more colloquial term for "testicles.") Several of the grizzled veterans of doping control nodded "yes."

My colleagues understood that the performance-enhancing benefits of testosterone would be very enticing to athletes. They worried that precedents such as this would tempt some athletes to falsely claim injuries in the expectation that they could then get a lasting advantage from a performance-enhancing drug they wouldn't otherwise be permitted to use.

In the end, we backed the young athlete's appeal. But when a lasting performance edge is likely, it's a tougher call, especially if there are decent alternatives or if the reduction in recovery time is small. The possibility that athletes will fake injuries or even induce them just to get a performance edge cannot be dismissed. Still, we have to leave the door open for instances in which the benefit to health is large, and the likelihood of a persistent advantage is small. In cases such as these, the TUE route, with all its imperfections, may be the most realistic way to balance the values at stake. If, on the other hand, convincing evidence emerges that a phenomenon such as "muscle memory"—the claim that the muscle-building impact of steroids lasts long after use is discontinued—is real, athletes and sports officials will have difficult choices to make.[18]

Commentators have tried to use the value of health both to condemn and to condone doping. A careful consideration of the arguments, and of the social forces shaping athletes' behavior, reinforces important insights. The ethics of performance-enhancing drug use depend on purpose, context, and consequences, not on the drug itself or on who happens to be using it. Permitting the use of PEDs by elite athletes is more likely to threaten their collective health than to protect it. Contagion to other groups, especially aspiring young athletes, is inevitable with a palpable risk of widespread harm. And, in the end, the ethics of PED use in sport depend on meanings, values, and the likely consequences for athletes' health.

NOTES

1. BBC News. Drugs stance stirs outrage. *BBC* [Internet]. 1998 Jul 27 [cited 2016 Aug 9]. Available from: http://news.bbc.co.uk/2/hi/sport/140315.stm.
2. Murray TH. The coercive power of drugs in sports. *Hastings Cent Rep.* 1983 Aug;13(4):24–30.
3. Sjoqvist F, Garle M, Rane A. Use of doping agents, particularly anabolic steroids, in sports and society. *Lancet.* 2008;371(9627):1872–1882.
4. Kayser B, Smith ACT. Globalisation of anti-doping: The reverse side of the medal. *BMJ.* 2008;337(7661):85–87.
5. Savulescu J, Foddy B, Clayton M. Why we should allow performance enhancing drugs in sport. *Br J Sports Med.* 2004 Dec;38(6):666–674.
6. US Food and Drug Administration. Press Announcements—FDA modifies dosing recommendations for Erythropoiesis-Stimulating Agents

[Internet]. 2011 [cited 2016 Aug 9]. Available from: http://www.fda.gov/NewsEvents/Newsroom/PressAnnouncements/ucm260670.htm.

7. Brio DL. Of MDs and muscles—lessons from two "retired steroid doctors." *JAMA J Am Med Assoc*. 1990 Mar 23;263(12):1697–1705.

8. Hoberman J. Sports physicians and the doping crisis in elite sport. *Clin J Sport Med*. 2002;12(4):203–208.

9. Waddington I, Smith A. *Sport, Health and Drugs: A Critical Sociological Perspective*. London; New York: Routledge; 2000. 228 p.

10. Gilbert B. Problems in a turned-on world. *Sports Illustrated*. 1969 Jun 23.

11. Hoberman J. Sports physicians and doping: Medical ethics and elite performance. In: Malcolm D and Safai, P editors. *The Social Organization of Sports Medicine: Critical Socio-Cultural Perspectives*. New York: Routledge; 2012. p. 247–264.

12. National Federation of State High School Associations. 2015–16 High School Athletics Participation Survey [Internet]. [cited 2017 Jan 2]. Available from: http://www.nfhs.org/ParticipationStatistics/PDF/2015-16_Sports_Participation_Survey.pdf.

13. Wiedeman R. A full revolution: In the run-up to the Olympics, Simone Biles is transforming gymnastics. [Internet]. *The New Yorker*. 2016 May 30 [cited 2016 Jul 6]. Available from: http://www.newyorker.com/magazine/2016/05/30/simone-biles-is-the-best-gymnast-in-the-world.

14. Savulescu J. Doping scandals, Rio and the future of human enhancement: Editorial. *Bioethics*. 2016 Jun;30(5):300–303.

15. Conte SA, Fleisig GS, Dines JS, Wilk KE, Aune KT, Patterson-Flynn N, et al. Prevalence of ulnar collateral ligament surgery in professional baseball players. *Am J Sports Med*. 2015 Jul 1;43(7):1764–1769.

16. Ahmad CS, Grantham WJ, Greiwe RM. Public perceptions of Tommy John surgery. *Phys Sportsmed*. 2012 May 1;40(2):64–72.

17. Bell, Stephania. What we've missed about Tommy John surgery [Internet]. ESPN.com. 2015 April 9 [cited 2016 Jun 20]. Available from: http://espn.go.com/mlb/story/_/id/12648769.

18. Gundersen K. Muscle memory and a new cellular model for muscle atrophy and hypertrophy. *J Exp Biol*. 2016 Jan 20;219(2):235–242.

Chapter 8

Is Anti-Doping Possible? Desirable? What Are the Alternatives?

Well, actually, in all honesty, that's what international track
meets are now.

Jamie Astaphan, MD, Ben Jonson's steroid supplier,
responding to a suggestion by Justice Dubin that we have a
separate contest between scientists,
pharmacologists, and doctors.

Giving athletes a fair chance of competing successfully while
competing clean is a tough assignment. You need to make it
easy to learn what's permitted and what's prohibited, including
implementing smart strategies for educating athletes. You need
methods to deter individuals who may be tempted to dope and
to detect those who cheat. And you need an adjudication system
that's fair with sanctions powerful enough to deter would-be
cheaters, but not draconian. Challenges arise at every step. Some
critics claim that the inescapable untidiness, the possibility of
errors, and the intrusiveness that comes with doping control are
reason enough to rethink how we deal with PEDs in sport. Other
critics urge abandoning all efforts to control them because,
they say, we are interfering with individuals' liberty to pursue
their own enhancement. Some go even further, arguing that
we should be applauding people's desire to improve themselves

with technologies of all kinds including performance-enhancing drugs instead of getting in their way.

There's an easy way to tell whether someone's objections are to the practical difficulties encountered by anti-doping or to the idea itself. Imagine that you were given a foolproof way to confirm whether an athlete had used a performance-enhancing drug. This marvelous method required no significant intrusion onto an athlete's body or privacy. No blood test. No urine sample. No "whereabouts" reporting. No "knock and pee" interruptions at home. Just a strand of hair. Imagine that from these tiny threads we could identify everyone who's using PEDs without falsely accusing innocent athletes.

This is, for the moment at least, a fantasy. But it's a useful way of clarifying the differences between the two main lines of attack against anti-doping. If we had a simple, cheap, and accurate detection method, many objections would fall away. Complaints about invasions of privacy, cost, and lab errors would disappear. But we're far from that now. These concerns are very much with us, as are the very real possibilities of corruption and injustice. The complaints about the practical difficulties encountered in anti-doping are the focus of this chapter.

AN UNSALVAGEABLE MESS?

My involvement in anti-doping began when Don Catlin, the dean of sport drug testing in the United States, heard me speak at a conference. I was soon asked to become a member of the USOC committee Don chaired that was charged with overseeing anti-doping. I continued in that role for more than a decade, meeting many interesting people along the way including bike road racer Connie Carpenter Phinney, who won Olympic gold in 1984 defeating a blood-doping teammate by the width of a rim, and Edwin Moses, the greatest hurdler of all time.

I'm grateful for the friendships formed, but working on these USOC committees was the most frustrating experience of my professional life. I couldn't escape the feeling that we were kept in the dark with no real opportunity to promote effective drug control. With one exception—Baaron Pittenger's time as Executive Director—I believe the USOC's leadership regarded any focus on doping as a nuisance, a distraction, and an impediment to fundraising. The athlete members of the committees, on the other hand, cared deeply. Athletes who don't dope, after all, are hurt most directly by those who do, and by ineffectual anti-doping programs.

I will have more to say about corruption, doping, and the governance of sport in chapter 9. First I want to consider complaints about the practice of anti-doping. Honoring the mantra "good ethics begins with good facts" means looking at the practical realities of anti-doping programs. It also means listening attentively to the voices of the people most directly affected: the athletes. Fortunately, we have some evidence of how athletes feel. Let's turn to the complaints about drug testing in practice.

PRIVACY, DECEIT, AND FAIRNESS

Given common ideas about bodily privacy, it's hard to imagine an athlete looking forward to peeing in full view of a drug control officer. Complying with the "whereabouts rules" that require informing anti-doping officials where you will be for an hour each day seems awfully constraining and intrusive. Both of these practices are significant invasions of individual's privacy, requiring good justification. It would matter a lot if athletes accepted them as necessary to assure fair competitions.

Doping control protocols typically require "observed voiding"—being watched while you pee to ensure that what goes into the sample jar was made by your kidneys and came from your bladder. Fake penises and bags of urine concealed in every imaginable orifice are not unheard of. Search online for clean urine and you'll find companies such as UrineTheClear (dial 877-REAL-PEE): For $60, plus shipping and handling, you can buy frozen or dehydrated urine guaranteed to pass a drug test. Or for $130 (on sale!), you could get a whizzinator— a fake penis filled with synthetic urine—in a choice of three colors.

Dan Hanley, a pioneer of anti-doping, told a story so good I fear it may be apocryphal—but I can't resist retelling it anyway. As Dan described the tale, the urine sample provided by a male athlete contained good news and bad news. The good news? No trace of banned drugs. The bad news? He was pregnant. More likely, he'd managed to substitute his girlfriend's urine for his own in the sample jar.

It might bother most people to be watched while we pee, but observed voiding does not appear to elicit strong or frequent complaints from athletes. Perhaps that's because they understand the lengths their doped competitors will go to avoid giving a valid sample. It's also possible that elite athletes can become so accustomed to other people's close attention to their bodies that the collector's gaze seems just more of the same.

The "whereabouts" requirement elicits more complaints. The current rule requires athletes to let testers know where they'll be for one hour each day between 5 a.m. and 11 p.m. so doping control officers can find them and obtain a sample.

Athletes complain that updating the information is a nuisance and that having to reveal their location violates their privacy. Missing three out-of-competition tests within twelve months because of inaccurate whereabouts information is considered a violation. If you're not doping and intentionally evading the sample collectors, you would have to be careless enough to fail to update your whereabouts multiple times, and unlucky enough to have testers look for you on at least three of those occasions.

The "whereabouts" system exists so that athletes can be tested while they're training, not just at events. Until out-of-competition testing began, athletes could and did use potent PEDs such as anabolic steroids and EPO between events; they just had to make certain by testing time that they were no longer "glowing"—the euphemism Tyler Hamilton and his teammates used for the interval during which their drug use was detectable. Without a whereabouts system and the ever-present threat of testing, doping athletes would be caught only if they goofed—if the "glow" was still visible in the sample they gave at the competition. In out-of-competition testing, doping control officials using the whereabouts information supplied by the athlete can show up within the appointed interval and demand a sample, meaning that all participating athletes are at risk of being tested on any given day.

Larry Bowers, former Chief Science Officer at the U.S. Anti-Doping Agency, explained that only a very small fraction of out-of-competition samples collected by USADA take place within that one-hour window. The vast majority of tests are done at other times of the day. If the athlete isn't available outside the specified one-hour window, there is no penalty for missing a test. But if the athlete is available, the doping control officer can request a sample. The aim of this practice is to reinforce the perception that the athlete could be tested at any time and thus to deter athletes from doping right after the window closes. Otherwise, twenty-three hours might be more than enough time for the "glow" to fade.

Based on his twenty-five years in anti-doping, Bowers sorts athletes into three groups in relation to doping. The "conformists" (his label) comprise roughly 40 percent of US athletes, he estimates. They support the rules against doping as correct and just and therefore will not cheat. The "deterrables," somewhere more than half of all athletes, might be susceptible to doping, but are responsive to education, testing, and other anti-doping programs. Finally come the "incorrigibles." In Larry's experience, this three to five percent of athletes don't respond to education or to deterrence. He believes they need to be caught and booted out of sport.

Scholars have criticized the whereabouts system, probably no one more severely than Lev Kreft: "Anti-doping measures apply to elite athletes to safeguard the clean trademark of the sport business, but they include a tendency to control all and everybody at any possible moment of their lives and whereabouts because these strengthen the grip of business over labour: even when you are a star of the first rank, you have to know who is really in charge."[1] (p160)

If we could pick up all doping athletes by testing at events, it's hard to imagine anyone willing to tolerate a whereabouts system or out-of-competition testing. But we're far from being able to do that at this time. A way to test Kreft's indictment is to see what athletes themselves say. In a survey about the impact on their daily lives, Danish athletes described what they disliked about whereabouts and out-of-competition testing. They talked about their fear of a warning, the feeling of surveillance, and the time it took from them. They also said it diminished the joy they found in sport. For all that, the same survey showed begrudging acceptance. Some athletes saw becoming subject to the whereabouts requirement as a kind of compliment—as recognition of their elite status.[2] Focus groups of US and Canadian athletes uncovered unanimous support. Indeed, these athletes wanted the testing to be "more stealth, less formulaic, more comprehensive (to include blood tests for example), and less predictable, in order to counter what is described in the current system as allowing for the potential of athletes to anticipate the procedures and thus circumvent the testing."[3] [(p13)] Not all feedback on the whereabouts system was so positive. A survey of Norwegian athletes conducted in the protocol's early days found worries that athletes in other nations were not subject to the same rigorous monitoring.[4] Strong majorities of elite Dutch athletes agreed that a whereabouts system was important in detecting and preventing doping, and necessary for a workable out-of-competition testing program. But many were unhappy with the intrusions on privacy of the current system, leading the authors to lament: "Sports policy is generally made for athletes, rarely in consultation with athletes, and almost never in partnership with athletes."[5]

On the whole, the available evidence suggests that athletes tolerate the whereabouts rules as an unwelcome but necessary nuisance. If they accept these measures, it's not because they're knuckling under to their bosses as Kreft claims, but because they understand that some of their competitors will dope if they can get away with it. The sooner we can replace the whereabouts requirement with something less intrusive, though, the better. And it's essential that athletes be full partners in evaluating and improving all aspects of anti-doping, including the whereabouts system.

IS THE LIGHT ANTI-DOPING SHINES WORTH THE CANDLE?

Is anti-doping worth its cost?[6,7] Many athletes evade detection. We know this from people such as Floyd Landis and Tyler Hamilton, who later admitted they used PEDs. Olympic sports federations now retest frozen samples gathered years ago. Improved lab methods continue to catch athletes whose samples slipped through earlier.

The people devising new drugs and new ways to avoid detection can be very clever. There is every reason to expect that the contest between athletes who dope on one side and the anti-doping agencies on the other will continue. Testing has had some successes. Many, including former dopers, regard the "biological passport" as a turning point. Rather than look for traces of prohibited substances, the biological passport establishes a physiological baseline for each athlete and looks for unusual patterns indicative of doping. Anti-doping organizations also are resorting more frequently to "non-analytical" methods—for example, investigations that rely on documents and testimony rather than test results. Lance Armstrong, in the end, was undone by overwhelming nonanalytical evidence that he'd led a sophisticated and ruthless doping program for his team rather than by a positive test.

Perspective is important. According to one accounting, the cost of anti-doping runs roughly between US$250 and US$500 million a year.[8] Of that total, WADA's annual budget is around US$30 million. Seems like a lot of money.

Consider, though, the economic value of sport. Estimates vary, but they agree that sport generates plenty of money. A.T. Kearney gauges the income from sports events—revenues from tickets, media rights, and sponsorships—at US$80 billion in

2014.[9] The international arm of PricewaterhouseCoopers added in the revenue from merchandizing and came up with a projected figure a tick over US$145 billion by 2015.[10] Anti-doping costs less than one-third of one percent of the total. Sport can afford to pay for first class anti-doping programs if it decides they're worth it.

Whether the money is well-spent is another question. If we agree that anti-doping is worthwhile in principle, we still have to ask if resources could be allocated more effectively and efficiently. Perhaps a larger share should go to education, research, or investigations rather than testing. A responsive and responsible organization will never cease asking how best to accomplish its mission and make adjustments accordingly.

JUSTICE AND INJUSTICE

Perfect justice in anti-doping would mean that everyone who knowingly benefited from PEDs would be caught and punished, and no one who did not would suffer sanctions. This leaves a third category: people whose performance has been enhanced, but without their knowledge or consent. The young girls swimming for East Germany at the height of that country's doping era likely fit this category. If we wished to do justice here, we could disqualify their records, but rather than sanction the athletes, we could seek to identify and punish the key actors in the ecosystem promoting doping: coaches, trainers, physicians, scientists, and officials.

The most common form of injustice in anti-doping comes from the failure to catch and sanction those who cheat. Some of this is the consequence of athletes outsmarting the system. But it also reflects the system's design. No imperfect human institution can achieve perfect justice, but you can choose which sort of errors you most want to avoid making. Sport has chosen to err on the side of not punishing the innocent, understanding that an unknown number of those who cheat will escape sanction.

The low rate of positive tests could mean that athletes are cheating and getting away with it. We know the denominator: the number of tests. We don't know the true numerator: the number of athletes using drugs. But we know it's higher than the number of positive tests, thanks to the many athletes who are eventually caught and confess to having used drugs for years despite never testing positive.

If a lab finds evidence of doping, the athlete's case is taken up by an adjudication system with different sport governing agencies, appellate bodies, and national courts. Most accused athletes protest their innocence, at least at first. Some ultimately acknowledge their drug use, a notable example being Floyd Landis, who had to surrender the yellow jersey worn by the winner of the Tour de France when traces of testosterone were found in his sample. He insisted for years that he'd raced clean, but then confessed and implicated other cyclists. Landis, though, turned out to be small potatoes compared to the most successful and notorious cheat in the Tour, Lance Armstrong.

If you want to defend an athlete against accusations of doping, by all means do so, but remember that protestations of innocence are the rule not the exception. Some critics of anti-doping leapt to defend the Danish bike racer Michael Rasmussen who'd been expelled from the Tour de France on what they asserted was "an allegation of doping (without evidence)."[11] Two years later Rasmussen admitted to doping from 1998 through 2010. He acknowledged using EPO, hGH, testosterone, DHEA, insulin, IGF-1, cortisone, and blood doping.[12]

Innocent athletes are sometimes charged with violating anti-doping rules. It's also possible that a positive test is the result of inadvertent ingestion of a banned drug. The test shows the presence of the substance, not how it got there. Some athletes protest that their positive test resulted from tainted food or nutritional supplements or from sabotage. Champion bike racer Alberto Contador blamed contaminated beef for the anabolic steroid clenbuterol found in his urine sample at the 2010 Tour de France. Greek 400-meter hurdles gold medalist Fani Halkia claimed that the steroid methyltrienolone in her sample must have come from a tampered dietary supplement. Halkia was one of fifteen Greek athletes found with that particular anabolic steroid, including eleven weightlifters in connection with the 2008 Beijing Olympic Games.[13] Both Contador and Halkia were banned from competition for two years.

Once a tainted sample is confirmed, the burden of proof rests on the athlete's shoulders. This "strict liability" provision is drummed into athletes, who are told that they are responsible for whatever they put into their body. Strict liability may seem to be a harsh standard. Without it, though, anti-doping agencies would have to prove not only the presence of a PED in the athlete's body but that the athlete knowingly took it with the intention of gaining a performance advantage. In practice, this would be an onerous burden of proof, rarely met. So "strict liability" remains the standard in anti-doping. If athletes can show there was no intent to dope, their sanction may be reduced.

HYPOXIC CHAMBERS, BLOOD DOPING, AND EPO: WHICH OF THESE THINGS IS NOT LIKE THE OTHERS?

Doping, at its core, means using drugs or other prohibited biomedical manipulations of an athlete's body to enhance performance. When athletes used blood transfusions to increase their endurance, it became known as "blood doping." More red blood cells transporting oxygen to starving muscles means being able to ride, run, or ski longer and harder. Some athletes can increase their red cells with a strategy known as "train low, live high." If you're able to live where the topography allows you to train near sea level but spend the remainder of your day and night in the clouds, the only technology you'd need is a car or perhaps a tram to take you high up the mountain. The net effect, if it works in your case, is a modest increase in red cell density and endurance. Most athletes are not so geographically favored, but if they live and train at low altitude, they can use a hypoxic chamber that allows them to sleep in an atmosphere of reduced oxygen equivalent to a mountaintop. Does that make the help of a hypoxic tent equivalent to taking EPO or blood doping? If EPO and blood doping are banned, must hypoxic chambers be banned as well? Or, if we allow hypoxic chambers, must we also permit blood doping and EPO?

Start with what we know about how each of these methods works. Blood doping directly and immediately increases the number of red cells in your blood. Once the body eliminates the excess fluid volume, what's left is an increased concentration of red cells. EPO works more slowly, stimulating your bone marrow to nudge blood stem cells onto the path that will transform them into red cells a couple of weeks later. (One way to pick up EPO use is to find an abnormal proportion of relatively young red cells.) Using an artificial hypoxic environment, on the other hand, stresses your cells, which increases production of a messenger molecule known as hypoxia-inducible factor 1 (HIF-1). HIF-1 has many effects, among them signaling your body to make more EPO, thereby launching the sequence for creating more red cells.

How dramatic and certain is the impact for each method? Blood doping is straightforward: Increasing your red cell concentration translates into a big boost in endurance. EPO takes longer to have its effect, but people close to elite sport claim enhancements in the range of 7 percent. One study claims the impact is not that dramatic.[14] Athletes' experience appears to favor the higher estimates; a single study to the contrary isn't enough to prove they're wrong.

The performance-enhancing impact of hypoxic chambers in "train low, live high" appears to be much less dramatic. A recent review of studies found improvements among elite athletes of around one percent.[15] A double-blinded placebo controlled study found no discernible impact on average.[16] That study found great variations in the way individuals responded to the strategy; it also found that the response may be "blunted" in elite athletes who are already near their red cell concentration maximum.

Deciding what differences ought to matter is a never-ending challenge for sport. Hypoxic chambers aren't exactly the same as transfusions or EPO. They work more slowly than transfusions. Their impact is highly variable, not terribly dramatic, and probably even less so in elite athletes who already are at peak fitness. And, unlike both transfusions and EPO, they don't short-circuit our body's normal physiological responses to intensive training. To the contrary: They depend on the stress of training to induce the complex array of responses that include making more red cells.

Loland and Hoppeler make the connection between training and what we value in sport:

> Biologically speaking, exercise training consists in using repeated stress of the organism to improve its performance under the specific stress conditions . . . Most substances

and methods on the doping list are qualitatively different because they bypass the body's natural and evolutionary based complex stress and compensation reactions. The use of prohibited substances and methods overruns natural talent, reduces athletes' possibilities of developing sporting excellence as human excellence in virtuous ways, and contradicts the spirit of sport . . . "[17] (p352)

A meeting held at WADA's Montreal headquarters to consider whether hypoxic chambers should be placed on the list of banned technologies proved to be a clarifying event. The case against permitting their use followed Loland's argument that to the extent a technology is administered and controlled by experts, it saps moral agency away from the athlete. The more an athlete's performance is the product of technologies overseen by such experts, the less the performance represents the combination of natural talent and its virtuous perfection at the core of the spirit of sport. The question was whether hypoxic chambers were contrary to the spirit of sport. It was noted that the athlete's part was essentially passive: sleeping in a chamber in which the oxygen concentration was artificially depleted.

One prominent sports scientist, a leading proponent of hypoxic chambers, objected to describing the athlete's role as passive. He insisted that recovery after intense training is far from a physiologically passive phenomenon. The body is going through a multitude of adaptations and processes. True enough. The scientist, though, was missing a crucial distinction, so I asked what we would think of an all-powerful king who decreed that anyone engaging in peristalsis would be summarily executed. Now, this anti-peristalsis tyrant is wrong in so many ways: cruel and capricious to begin with. But I was interested in a moral confusion evidenced in the tyrant's decree.

When your stomach rumbles, you're experiencing the audible evidence of peristalsis—an involuntary constriction of your intestines. Punishing someone in whom peristalsis is happening, or praising or rewarding them for it, makes no sense. We can't control it, and it happens to everyone. At the same time, just like recovery from training, peristalsis is an active, vital physiological process. From the standpoint of physiology, then, recovery from training is indeed active not passive. But the relevant standpoint for deciding whether hypoxic chambers undermined the spirit of sport was ethics, not physiology. Lying in bed while the magic happens is, morally speaking, more passive than active.

Only later did I realize that the advocate had a better argument available in defense of the hypoxic devices. We could have taken a wider view. Spending the night sleeping in one of these devices after a sluggish day likely won't provide much, if any, benefit in the form of enhanced endurance. What value the strategy has for improving performance requires the "train low" half of the "train low, live high" program. The athlete must train hard in order to benefit from artificially "sleeping high." Dedicated training is an essential part of what we value in the spirit of sport. It's a component of the virtuous perfection of a person's natural talents. From a wider view, then, hypoxic chambers used in concert with intense training seem far more like post-workout massages or meticulous attention to nutrition and health than physiological shortcuts such as EPO or transfusions.

An advantage of hard cases such as hypoxic chambers is that they force us to say what really matters. What should we ask of athletes? What sacrifices should we expect them to make? What risks should we encourage them to take? How much control over their lives should be given to experts who prod, poke, demand, and manipulate? Should athletes become ever more the instruments through which other actors—coaches, trainers, doping gurus—exercise their dominion? Should sport serve the larger interests of athletes, or is maximum performance through whatever means all that matters?

The discussion at WADA that day made it clear that the athletes and sports scientists present felt strongly that "train low/ live high" with the help of hypoxic chambers was much more similar to other training strategies than it was to taking anabolic steroids or EPO. If you believe, as I do, that we should listen to athletes, the right decision was clear: Permit hypoxic devices— but, at the same time, keep a watchful eye on expert-controlled technologies' impact on athletes' lives. This is not the kind of problem that can be solved once and for all; rather, it's an enduring tension we must continue to monitor attentively.

LIBERTARIANISM, TRANSHUMANISM, AND THE FUTURE OF SPORT

The criticisms so far in this chapter focus on imperfections in implementing anti-doping. They don't deny that keeping at least some PEDs out of sport can have a legitimate purpose. Imagine that we had the test I described at the beginning of this chapter. A strand of hair recovered at a time and place convenient for the athlete and voila! We'd know who had used a performance-enhancing drug. This marvelous method, though, wouldn't sway anti-doping critics who embrace enhancing humans as positive and good in itself. Some thinkers celebrate technologies that enhance human performance in sport and in other realms of human life as expressions of our ingenuity, creativity, and will. (Attentive readers will note that at times I refer to criticisms, at other times to critics. The criticisms are often very different in their significance for the future of sport. Critics of anti-doping, however, tend to borrow freely from the full range of criticisms.) Critics differ in how much importance they assign to fairness in sport, but many proclaim that technologies of enhancement will make sport more rather than less fair. At the further reaches of the movement that calls itself Transhumanism, the vision is to transcend human limitations: to enhance our minds, expand our consciousness, improve and immortalize our bodies. Imagine future athletes whose bodies are transformed chemically, genetically, and surgically, with new powers, possibly merged with machines or computers, capable of feats unimaginable with the all-too-human bodies of even the most superb athletes today.

The enhancements these writers imagine go far beyond sport. I believe there are lessons in our experience with performance-enhancing technologies in sport that can help us deal sensibly and wisely with promises of technological enhancement in other realms of human life as well. We'll look at those lessons in the next and final chapter along with the need for credible reform in the way sport governs itself. Only then can athletes be confident that doping is not tilting the playing field.

NOTES

1. Kreft L. Elite sportspersons and commodity control: Anti-doping as quality assurance. *Int J Sport Policy Polit.* 2011 Jul;3(2):151–161.
2. Overbye M, Wagner U. Experiences, attitudes and trust: An inquiry into elite athletes' perception of the whereabouts reporting system. *Int J Sport Policy Polit.* 2013 May;6(3):1–22.
3. Johnson J, Butryn T, Masucci M. A focus group analysis of the US and Canadian female triathletes' knowledge of doping. *Sport Soc.* 2013 Jun;16(5):654–671.
4. Hanstad DV, Skille EÅ, Thurston M. Elite athletes' perspectives on providing whereabouts information: A survey of athletes in the Norwegian registered testing pool. *Sport Soc.* 2009;6(1):30–46.

5. Valkenburg D, de Hon O, van Hilvoorde I. Doping control, providing whereabouts and the importance of privacy for elite athletes. *Int J Drug Policy*. 2014;25(2):212–218.
6. Kayser B, Mauron A, Miah A. Viewpoint: Legalisation of performance-enhancing drugs. *Lancet*. 2005;366 Suppl:S21.
7. Kayser B, Mauron A, Miah A. Current anti-doping policy: A critical appraisal. *BMC Med Ethics*. 2007;8(2):1–10.
8. Maennig W. Inefficiency of the anti-doping system: Cost reduction proposals. *Subst Use Misuse*. 2014 Jul 29;49(9):1201–1205.
9. ATKearney LLC. Winning in the business of sport [Internet]. 2014. Available from: https://www.atkearney.com/documents/10192/5258876/Winning+in+the+Business+of+Sports.pdf/ed85b644-7633-469d-8f7a-99e4a50aadc8.
10. pwc.com/sports outlook. Changing the game: Outlook for the global sports market to 2015 [Internet]. 2011 Dec. Available from: http://www.pwc.com/gx/en/hospitality-leisure/pdf/changing-the-game-outlook-for-the-global-sports-market-to-2015.pdf.
11. Savulescu J, Foddy B. Le Tour and failure of zero tolerance: Time to relax doping controls. In: Savulescu J, ter Meulen R, Kahane G, editors. *Enhancing Human Capacities*. Oxford: Wiley Blackwell; 2011. p. 304–312.
12. Stokes S. Michael Rasmussen retires and admits doping over a fourteen year timeframe [Internet]. *Velonation*. 2013 Jan 31 [cited 2016 Nov 23]. Available from: http://www.velonation.com/News/ID/13829/Michael-Rasmussen-retires-and-admits-doping-over-a-fourteen-year-timeframe.aspx.
13. Associated Press. Greek federation suspends Halkia two years for doping [Internet]. *ESPN.com*. 2008 Nov 27 [cited 2016 Jul 5]. Available from: http://espn.go.com/olympics/trackandfield/news/story?id=3730257.
14. Lodewijkx HFM, Brouwe B, Kuipers H, Hezewijk R van. Overestimated effect of EPO Administration on aerobic exercise capacity: A meta-analysis. *Am J Sports Sci Med*. 2013;1(2):17–27.
15. Sinex JA, Chapman RF. Hypoxic training methods for improving endurance exercise performance. *J Sport Health Sci*. 2015 Dec;4(4):325–332.
16. Siebenmann C, Robach P, Jacobs RA, Rasmussen P, Nordsborg N, Diaz V, et al. "Live high–train low" using normobaric hypoxia: A double-blinded, placebo-controlled study. *J Appl Physiol*. 2011 Dec 21;112(1):106–117.
17. Loland S, Hoppeler H. Justifying anti-doping: The fair opportunity principle and the biology of performance enhancement. *Eur J Sport Sci*. 2012;12(4):347–353.

Chapter 9

On the Meaning and Future of Sport

[A]fter a game one often says that the losing side deserved to win. Here one does not mean that the victors are not entitled to claim the championship, or whatever spoils go to the winner. One means instead that the losing team displayed to a higher degree the skills and qualities that the game calls forth, and the exercise of which gives the sport its appeal. Therefore the losers truly deserved to win but lost out as a result of bad luck, or from other contingencies that caused the contest to miscarry.

John Rawls

Two crucial challenges remain for the future of sport. One is self-inflicted. The governance of sport often has been weak, sometimes corrupt, and in general disinclined to provide anti-doping the independence and the resources it needs to be effective. The second challenge is to the idea that sport should value "natural talents" at all; in its place, it envisions a merging of people and technology to achieve performances far beyond the capacities of today's human bodies and minds.

In preparing to tackle these two challenges, it's worth reflecting on the approach I've taken and to summarize what has been established so far. The method is more "bottom up" than "top down." I didn't begin with a grand philosophical theory of sports ethics, but instead stuck close to the ground. Thoughtful decisions about rules and equipment brought out particular values and meanings latent in sport. Those values and meanings, in turn, have profound implications for the ethics of doping. We also tested these ideas against the toughest challenges posed by prominent critics of anti-doping.

The Hastings Center, the pioneering bioethics research institute so important in shaping my approach, has a mantra: "good ethics begins with good facts." In the case of drugs in sport, that meant delving into the science of sport performance enhancement and the practical challenges to anti-doping. By far the most important revelation was the relentless competitive dynamic that drives many athletes to dope. The voices of elite athletes in chapter 1 make it clear that in the absence of effective, trustworthy anti-doping programs, they faced three bad options: compete at a disadvantage and probably lose to those using PEDs; give up competing at the level that your talents and dedication deserve; or give in and dope like your competitors.

Some claims by anti-doping critics weren't hard to rebut. For example, the notion that athletes are making completely free, autonomous choices whether to dope falls apart once we appreciate the dynamic that impels athletes never to surrender a competitive advantage. Some individuals may indeed freely choose to dope. Their decisions have inexorable consequences for their fellow athletes. In that unyielding environment, allowing some athletes to dope means in effect that every athlete hoping to be successful feels compelled to do the same. This is why I describe doping in the context of elite sport as "tyrannical." Add to this relentless dynamic the specter of athlete ecosystems—coaches, trainers, sports officials, even national governments—encouraging, facilitating, sometimes imposing, and covering up doping, and the myth of the athlete-philosopher calmly and dispassionately weighing the pros and cons of doping is exposed as the fantasy it is for most elite athletes.

Anti-doping critics also offered more serious challenges. One common suggestion is to "level the playing field" by letting all athletes dope. Setting aside for the moment the public health implications of opening the PED floodgates, the critics have a point. If everyone had access to the same PEDs, competitions would not be unfair in that respect. Responding to this challenge required a deeper inquiry into meaning and values in sport.

I don't want to overwhelm readers with philosophical detail. I hope it's enough to say that the method used in this inquiry is inspired by John Rawls's reflective equilibrium, moving back and forth from close observations of what sport appears to care about to more abstract generalizations. If successful, it results in " . . . identifying a framework of value implicit in a sphere of human endeavor and then determining what the moral nature of a person must be in order for them to find value in such a sphere."[1] (p180), [2] My goal was to describe the meanings and values embedded in sport in a manner that would be consistent and intelligible to people knowledgeable about the practice of sport. An insightful account also would help identify the factors shaping justice and injustice in the sphere of human endeavor we call sport.[3]

My inquiries into meaning and values yielded an account of what we care about in sport: excellent performance as the joint product of natural talents and the dedication required to perfect those talents. Add to that the courage to perform under pressure, and I believe we have a description that people who participate in, love, and understand sport will recognize.

Chapter 2 acknowledged that natural talents are not earned or deserved; they just are. The talents that make for success in different sports vary widely, and may have little to do with leading a worthwhile life outside of sport. The virtues required to perfect those talents, on the other hand, like self-discipline, teamwork, and perseverance, are earned and are relevant across all sports and throughout all spheres of life.

The talents enabling success in sport are not distributed equally. Some critics argue that inherited differences in people's athletic talents should be compensated for by PEDs or genetic enhancements. But when it comes to athletic gifts, unequal is not the same as unfair. And neither PEDs nor genetic enhancement likely will succeed in leveling out differences in natural talents anyway.

One way to learn what a sport cares about is to look at its rules, in particular how those rules adapt to changes in technology, strategies, and the players themselves. By tracing responses to several such challenges, chapter 3 revealed useful insights: First, every sport needs rules that reflect what it values; second, good rules strive to minimize the influence of factors apart from those that sport believes ought to matter; and third, in every sport, the factors making decisive differences should be the natural talents that sport values coupled with the dedication needed to perfect those talents.

Creating level playing fields for Paralympic athletes—with ten distinct categories of impairments, some with multiple degrees of severity—requires paying particularly close attention to values and meanings in sport, as chapter 4 showed. The Paralympics have had to be explicit about the factors that should influence athletic success and about what counts as a fair competition. From prosthetic limbs to wheelchairs and throwing frames, technology plays a vital role in enabling many parathletes to compete at all. The International Paralympic Committee insists that talent and dedication should be decisive, so it requires that advantageous enabling technologies should be available to all competitors—and that performance-enhancing drugs should be banned.

Geography, climate, economics, and family resources are among the many circumstances that influence whether a person's athletic talents are noticed and nurtured. Chapter 5 argued that although differences in circumstances are ubiquitous and not unfair in themselves, sport should address differences *in access to* competitions by expanding opportunities to develop each individual's talents. In no case, however, should sport tolerate discrimination of any kind against athletes. Unfairness *in competition*, likewise, undermines what is valuable and meaning ful in sport and should never be tolerated.

Gender is an especially fraught issue for sport. Women often have been treated poorly in Olympic sports. Women whose gender identity was questioned have had an especially rough time of it. Chapter 6 addressed the quandary posed by women with high natural amounts of testosterone and the advantages in strength and power that come with it. These women are not doping. But women without those hormonal advantages also deserve a level playing field. Sport's challenge is to devise policies that provide all women a fair chance to compete. At the same time, sport must be respectful of the privacy and gender identity of women whose performance may be benefiting from male levels of muscle-building hormones. The same values and meanings that guide sport's policies on PEDs should shape policy on gender and eligibility. Recent cases demonstrate how difficult that can be to do well.

Chapter 7 looked critically at how the concept of health has been used in the debate over doping. On the one hand, it's clear that the ethics of performance-enhancing drug use depend on purpose, context, and consequences, not on the drug itself or on who happens to be using it. A drug banned from competitions may be helpful, even irreplaceable, for treating disease or recovering from injury and therefore permitted under appropriate circumstances. Nevertheless, permitting the widespread use of PEDs by elite athletes more likely will threaten their health than protect it. Should the ban on PEDs ever be lifted, contagion to other groups, especially aspiring young athletes, seems inevitable with a risk of widespread harm.

SPORT GOVERNANCE AND ANTI-DOPING

Chapter 8 tackled complaints about the practical difficulties encountered in executing an anti-doping program. However, the best science, sharpest labs, and most-skilled sample collectors in the world aren't enough on their own. For athletes to have confidence they can compete clean and have a fair shot at winning, the organizations that govern sport must prove they are reliable, competent, and free from corruption. Recent events demonstrate we have some distance to travel before we reach that goal. Corruption and exploitation, sadly, are all too common.

Beginning in the 1960s, East Germany launched a sophisticated, state-sponsored doping operation. Girl swimmers of fourteen and younger were given powerful anabolic steroids. Fourteen- and fifteen-year-old girls and boys competing in canoeing, kayaking, and other sports received the same. In October 1974, a "Top Secret" bill was passed that organized doping centrally and made it integral to preparation for important international competitions. The bill called for research to optimize doping, instruction for physicians and coaches, and absolute secrecy about the entire program. Young female swimmers from East Germany dominated the Olympics in that era, which that

country touted as evidence of the superiority of its political system—the same system whose collapse has become synonymous
with the destruction in 1989 of the wall dividing East and West
Berlin.[4]

Olympic officials' inability to mount a credible attack on doping was obvious enough by the year 2000 to spur the creation
of the World Anti-Doping Agency.[5] Many years later, despite
progress, major problems remain. The list of sport organizations
accused of indifference or outright fraud and corruption around
doping continues to grow.

My current role as a member of the IAAF Ethics Board provided a glimpse into the contemporary culture of doping in
Russia. Lilya Shobukova was a very successful long distance
runner who won the Chicago marathon three times and the
London marathon once. Success on that scale translates to
lucrative appearance fees and prize money. Shobukova tested
positive but escaped sanction for two years because, as she
testified, she and her husband paid blackmail to two senior
Russian sports officials and their co-conspirators, including
IAAF's head of anti-doping and a son of the then-IAAF president. When, eventually, she was sanctioned, the Shobukovas
demanded repayment of the 450,000 Euros they'd paid. By
their account, just 300,000 were returned, and they went public with their accusations. Shobukova's complaint was that the
blackmailers did not keep their promise. (A deal's a deal, I suppose.) The Board's investigation led to charges of violations of
the IAAF Ethics Code against four individuals. The Ethics Board
hearing panel had an opportunity to question Shobukova and
her husband, three of the four accused parties, and witnesses.
It seemed to me as a member of the hearing panel that the people accused of blackmailing Shobukova to cover up her doping
regarded it as business as usual.[6]

Since then, more evidence has emerged. The WADA Independent Commission investigating reports of doping in Russian athletics reported it had found a "deeply rooted culture of cheating."[7] [(p22)] Investigators found evidence that ARAF, the All-Russian Athletics Federation, was exploiting its athletes with the collusion of doctors, coaches, and lab personnel. Part 2 of the Commission's report, which appeared after our Ethics Board judgment was posted, found further evidence of corruption and bribery at IAAF implicating its former President, Lamine Diack.[8] This report describes how Diack used his position at IAAF to hire two of his sons as "consultants" along with a "presidential legal advisor." In this way he ". . . created a close inner circle, which filtered and funneled communications to and from senior IAAF staff, ultimately functioning as an informal illegitimate governance structure outside the formal IAAF governance structure."[8] [(p4)]

Around this time, two individuals who had served as senior staff members at Russia's Moscow anti-doping lab died suddenly and unexpectedly just as the lab came under suspicion for complicity in facilitating doping by Russian athletes. An independent investigator charged by WADA to look further into allegations of cover-ups by the lab at the Sochi Winter Games found that, "The Ministry of Sport directed, controlled and oversaw the manipulation of athlete's analytical results or sample swapping, with the active participation and assistance of the FSB (Russian Federal Security Service), CSP (Center of Sports Preparation for Russian National Teams), and both Moscow and Sochi Laboratories."[9] [(p86)]

A follow-up report provided further evidence of the elaborate conspiracy to provide PEDs to Russian athletes while shielding them from consequences. The Moscow lab informed the Ministry of Sport of more than 1231 positive samples that never were disclosed to the international drug control authorities. The lab perfected a "disappearing positive methodology," becoming what the report describes as "the vital final cog in a much larger machine that enabled athletes to compete while using PEDs and resulted in unprecedented cheating within the doping control mechanism in Russia."[10 (p53)] Massive, systemic cheating began years before the Sochi Winter Olympics. The second McLaren report notes: "The Russian Olympic team corrupted the London Games 2012 on an unprecedented scale, the extent of which will probably never be fully established."[10 (p77)] The report's verdict on the conspirators' ethics is, if anything, too mild: "The desire to win medals superseded their collective moral and ethical compass and Olympic values of fair play."[10 (p78)]

Athletes and sports officials from other countries, along with leaders in the international anti-doping movement, including the World Anti-Doping Agency, called for a ban on all Russian athletes from the 2016 Rio Olympics, making exceptions for only those who had been tested extensively outside of Russia with no positive tests. The IOC, however, balked at a blanket ban of Russian athletes, instead leaving it to each international federation to decide, leading to nasty exchanges between officials with WADA and the IOC. Many athletes, always wary of competing against those who dope, were not happy when Russians competed against them in Rio.

Did the IOC's decision show a lack of nerve? Did it demonstrate the political power and connections of Russian officials? Or was it a nuanced response to Russian athletes who may not have doped but would have been punished by a general ban? What I don't see reflected at all in the IOC's decision is concern for those athletes who do not dope and hate losing to those who do. Those have always been the people I worry about most.

To be fair, it's not just one country. Kenyan sports officials have been accused of demanding bribes from their athletes to cover up doping positives. Other nations have had their scandals, including the United States, and more surely will come to light.

GOVERNANCE, INDEPENDENCE, AND THE FUTURE OF SPORT

Successful anti-doping efforts require more than competent labs and sample collectors. They need independence, sturdy safeguards against corruption, and a sophisticated understanding of how institutions function. Historically, a sport's international federation or national Olympic body would establish—and control—its own anti-doping program. The federations and national Olympic committees are accustomed to governing themselves. Who better, after all, to decide what rules should govern swimming or weightlifting than the people who know their sport best?

Anti-doping is different. International federations have commercial and reputational interests in avoiding doping scandals. They benefit when attractive star athletes emerge: more coverage, popularity, and money for their sport. The last thing they want is for their stars to be exposed as cheats. Likewise with national Olympic committees, who may be expected to demonstrate their country's superiority by running up the medal count.

It's long past time to acknowledge the conflicts of interest created when organizations and individuals that profit from a sport also control its anti-doping programs. Allowing powerful conflicting interests to go unremarked and unmanaged hasn't worked well in other settings; there's no reason to think it fares any better in sport. National and international sports bodies must ensure that anti-doping authorities are trustworthy, independent entities, not subject to undue influence. Just as corporations and nonprofits must subject themselves to independent audits of their finances, so the integrity of competitions depends on anti-doping's independence from the institutions that benefit from that sport.

The urgent need to assure integrity extends far beyond anti-doping. With vast amounts of money and prestige at stake, far too many officials have yielded to temptations to take advantage of their positions. It's not that people have ignored the need for good governance in sport organizations. An abundance of reports, studies, and guidance documents brim with good ideas and wonderful-sounding principles such as transparency, accountability, independence, equity, and democracy. What's lacking is the will to make the necessary reforms over the opposition of entrenched forces who stand to lose —or be exposed—if genuine reform succeeds.

The aura of virtue, talent, and effort that envelopes sport provides cover for grifters eager to take advantage. International sport needs a revolution in governance. The organizations that oversee Olympic sports must be accountable and should serve the interests and welfare of athletes, not the greater glory and the bank accounts of those entrusted with running them.

SPORT, TECHNOLOGY, AND WHAT IT MEANS TO BE HUMAN

Blackmail, bribery, and corruption are threats to the future of sport that don't require subtle balancing or philosophical analysis. They're wrong, period. Another challenge to the future of sport, however, is philosophical to the core: It imagines athletes of the future as creatures in which technologies merge with human bodies in pursuit of spectacular performances we can scarcely imagine today. The contrast with the conception of sport at the heart of this book—the virtuous perfection of *natural* talents—is sharp and clear.

Whatever else it does, sport affirms our connection to our physical body. I've wondered whether as our lives become increasingly devoted to screens—smartphones, tablets, computers, televisions—our physical bodies seem to diminish in significance. In our work and our leisure, they can become nuisances. Bodies need to be fed and watered. They grow weary. They need rest. They distract us from where we desire to focus our attention.

There are notable exceptions, of course. Meals can be an occasion for physical pleasure and social interaction. My mother was Italian. Her parents emigrated from the Abruzzo region in Italy to Philadelphia. They brought with them a love of good food. Preparing and sharing delicious meals was an important way my Italian family showed its love. Not everyone thinks of food that way. To Rob Rhinehart, a tech entrepreneur, feeding himself was an expensive nuisance. He decided that he could save money and time by mixing thirty-five nutrients into a slurry he calls Soylent. It's now a hundred-million-dollar business. Referring to a poster showing metabolic pathways, he told an interviewer, "This is life—a walking chemical reaction."[11] Of course, food doesn't have to be an either/or choice. You can enjoy feasts with people you love, and still grab something fast and convenient when other things feel more important. In making these choices, you are declaring what you value, and, perhaps without any conscious deliberation, you are shaping your life in accordance with those values and meanings.

Sex, happily, still requires your physical body. And then there is sport. Sport celebrates physical excellence as shaped and perfected by intentional activity. When we train, our will and our body are in a kind of harmony—or at least begrudging collaboration. Success in sport demands intimate cooperation between our often-recalcitrant physical body and our will that coaxes, demands work and sacrifice, and sustains a vision of goals to be achieved. Sport connects our capacity as moral agents with our embodiment as finite biological creatures.

The Norwegian philosopher Sigmund Loland has written thoughtfully about the relationship of technology, expertise, and moral agency in sport. He encourages us to understand technology as "human-made means to reach human interests and goals."[12 (p153)] Sport makes use of technologies of all kinds, but Loland singles out for special concern biomedical technologies that enhance performance. The problem with what he calls "expert-administrated" technologies is that "they are designed to enhance performance without really requiring athlete effort and control."[12 (p155)] The athlete's moral agency is limited to seeking, or merely acquiescing to, experts' authority over their bodies. This is only a problem if we believe that sport should value athletes' dedication and perseverance. Not all ideas about the meaning of sport share that belief.

TECHNOLOGY AND VALUES IN SPORT

Loland describes three conceptions of technology and values in sport. The first, *sportive relativism,* couldn't care less about intrinsic values or meaning in sport; what matters in sportive relativism is how much sport contributes to other goals, such as nationalism, ideology, entertainment, or profit. Deciding whether to employ a performance-enhancing technology becomes a purely instrumental question: Does it improve the entertainment value of our product and increase our profits? Does it demonstrate the superiority of our nation or political system? The massive Russian doping and cover-up at the 2014 Sochi Winter Games likely was motivated by the desire to reinforce Russian nationalism and boost the government's popularity. That was manifestly true of East Germany's state-run doping program. Sportive relativism may not be philosophically enlightening or interesting, but it remains a powerful influence on sport and therefore deserves to be noted.

Loland dubs the second idea the "narrow theory," which holds that the ultimate goal of sport is maximizing human performance. Oxford philosopher Julian Savulescu and colleagues wrote this about the meaning of sport: "In many ways the athletic ideal of modern athletes is inspired by the myth of the marathon. Their ideal is superhuman performance, at any cost."[13] (p666) They acknowledge that the marathon runner in the classic tale dropped dead.

Proponents of the narrow theory have little patience with ideas about natural talents or quibbles over technologies that improve performance. The goal in the narrow theory is to break the record. If a drug or genetic tweak can help, so be it. They acknowledge no intrinsic values within sport significant enough to constrain the quest for ever-improved results. People who think otherwise are dismissed as "bioconservatives" who aren't sufficiently optimistic about what technology can do for us, and paternalists for placing obstacles in the way of athletes who want to use performance-enhancing drugs.

Loland calls the third conception the "wide theory." The wide theory has certain traits in common with each of the other conceptions. It shares with sportive relativism the assumption that sport is deeply connected with larger goals. But it refuses to see sport as always and only an instrument to other ends. The wide theory agrees with the narrow view that we can find values and meanings within sport. But it insists that those values and meanings are much broader and diverse than the narrow view's single-minded focus on maximizing performance. To the contrary, in the wider theory, sport's values and meanings are intertwined with other vital human institutions and ideals. Sport can help societies to thrive and contribute to the flourishing of individuals. The wide theory's attitude toward technology is grounded in a nuanced account of values and meanings in sport. Loland writes: "In contradistinction to the narrow theory, the wide theory accepts regulations of biomedical means and methods. Athletes are to realize their potential as moral agents and this can only be achieved if they have insight in, control over and responsibility for their performance."[12 (p158)]

Loland and I—along with McNamee, Simon and other scholars—represent this wider view. I believe that technologies that improve performance have their place in sport, but they must be measured against whatever unwanted impact they have on sport's meaning and values. Technology is suspect if it diminishes athletes' moral agency, relocates control to experts, or otherwise undermines the connections among talent, dedication, and performance. Anabolic steroids, EPO, and other performance-enhancing drugs fail this test.

Of course, athletes work closely with coaches, trainers, and sports scientists without evoking worries about excessive expert control. What's the difference? Consider what coaches do. For example, they teach techniques and strategy. I taught the rudiments of the 1-3-1 zone press to a grade-school basketball team I coached in a North Philadelphia parochial school while I was a student at Temple University. My twelve- to fourteen-year-old players could run and jump, but they had no idea how to collaborate as a team. I decided to build a strategy around their energy and aggressiveness. In the 1-3-1 press, the opposing player receiving the inbounds pass immediately found two of our players on top of him. Their assignment was to harass the ball-handler with the intent of forcing a hurried pass or stealing the ball. If the other team threw the ball up the court, our remaining defenders tried to intercept it. (It helped that long passes sometimes deflected off our gym's low ceiling.) Once our players had the ball, they were supposed to drive to the basket for a layup. I recall a game when our most athletic player stole the ball and darted toward the basket just as we'd practiced—only to dribble to the corner and launch a fall-away jump shot. It wasn't pretty, and their coach—me—wasn't capable of teaching them anything more sophisticated. But it worked well enough for our team to win every game that season except one— against a Catholic orphanage with an impressive gym and players who had plenty of time to practice and, I'm sure, a much better coach.

When athletes learn from good coaches and train for countless hours to improve themselves, each athlete remains the author of his or her own performance. A successful competitor may credit coaches, teammates, parents, or God, but that athlete's particular talent, honed through perseverance and dedication, plays an indispensable role in whatever is admirable and successful in that performance. When athletes decide to "install" capacity— say increasing endurance with injections of EPO—they are morally responsible for such decisions, but it's not something to be admired as a virtuous perfection of natural talents. It requires no more talent or effort than what's required to use a syringe.

TRANSHUMANIST VISIONS

A passage from Nick Bostrom's imaginary "Letter from Utopia" conveys the flavor of Transhumanist thought: "You could say

I am happy, that I feel good. You could say that I feel surpassing bliss. But these are words invented to describe human experience. What I feel is as far beyond human feelings as my thoughts are beyond human thoughts. I wish I could show you what I have in mind. If only I could share one second of my conscious life with you!"[14] (p3) The "letter" is signed "Your Possible Future Self."

Transhumanists and their philosophical brethren embrace technologies that modify the human body. The Transhumanist movement celebrates such modifications as expressions of human creativity and imagination. Transhumanists, interestingly, tend to be men rather than women, although there are notable exceptions such as Natasha Vita-More, who described her desired "eclectic look" suitable for a party: ". . . a glistening bronze skin with emerald green highlights, enhanced height to tower above other people, a sophisticated internal sound system so that I could alter the music to suit my own taste, memory enhance device, emotional-select for feel-good people so I wouldn't get dragged into anyone's inappropriate conversations. And parabolic hearing so that I could listen in on conversations across the room if the one I was currently in started winding down."[15] (p517)

Transhumanists have ambitions far beyond the playing fields of Eton—or Fenway Park, the Birds Nest Stadium in Beijing, or the cross-country ski trails of Oslo. They want to redefine and remake humankind in keeping with their vision of human bodies and minds merging with technology. Applying their ideas to sport offers some insights into the implications of their larger project. Andy Miah, for example, urges us to embrace a future "where everyone is free to choose the enhancements that best accentuate their performance. That is what the natural athlete should look like today . . . let us celebrate the rise of a new age of genuinely superhuman athletes, where the rules of sports are governed not by ever-present but ultimately unreliable doping police, but by a genuine concern for optimizing excellence. As technology gets better, athletes should, too."[16]

I understand the optimism and enthusiasm surrounding technology. As an avid reader of science fiction in my youth and a close follower of science all my adult life, I appreciate what technology has done to improve lives. But technology and science can never tell us what deserves to be valued or how to build a rich, meaningful life. Miah's call for technologically enhanced athletes isn't wrong in itself, though we do need to pay attention to the risks to the individual; we also need to assure that the ripples from it don't damage other important values.

The problem for sport is what I've dubbed the libertarian enhancement quandary, which goes roughly like this: My liberty to use whatever enhancement technologies I desire has at least two unfortunate consequences. First, to the extent that I must surrender control to experts administering these technologies, my moral agency is diminished. I remain responsible for the consequences of my choice, of course, but I don't deserve full credit for whatever athletic achievements result from the experts' manipulations. Second, in the competitive context of sport, performance-enhancing technologies are tyrannical. To the extent they're effective, if some athletes use them other athletes must do the same to remain competitive. The option of competing successfully without PEDs or similar technologies fades in direct proportion to the technology's impact on performance. Exercising my free choice to use PEDs exerts powerful coercive pressures on the choices of others.

I want to defend a conception of sport free from domination by performance-enhancing technologies—the domination that would inevitably follow if PEDs were allowed. People such as the

Transhumanists are free, of course, to pursue alternative visions. It's their right to advocate for a world competition that welcomes performance-enhancing technologies of all kinds. Perhaps a Global Transhumanist Games would command the world's interest with its astounding new record feats while the Olympic Games fade into obscurity. I believe that would be a loss, but the people of the future may not agree or care. Or perhaps the two events could survive side by side, the way powerlifting with its rigid shirts and, in some versions, indifference to doping, exists alongside Olympic weightlifting.[17]

My aim in this book is to show that sport is rich in values and meanings worth preserving and, further, that incorporating doping and other technological enhancements into sport would irrevocably undermine those values and meanings. Whether you think they are worth protecting is up to you. Preserving the possibility of competitions without doping would allow us to continue to marvel at natural talents and to admire the dedication needed to perfect them.

THE CONCEPT OF "NATURAL TALENTS" AND ITS PRACTICAL APPLICATION IN SPORT

The Transhumanist alternative would show us what the merger of human bodies and technology can achieve. Transhumanism doesn't seem to find much value in the concept of "natural talents." The movement is more inclined to bemoan the limitations imposed by our physical body and brain and seek to overcome them with technologies. What then can we make of sport's celebration of natural talents?

The significance of natural talents emerged through the details of sport's efforts to grapple with a series of challenges: New equipment such as bamboo vaulting poles, whole-body swimsuits and hinged speedskates; new competitors such as parathletes in wheelchairs and seven-foot-tall basketball players. Whenever a sport has to decide what differences should be allowed to make a difference, it must reflect on the sources of its meaning and value. These self-examinations seem always to embrace natural talents and the dedication needed to perfect those talents as sources of value and meaning.

Not surprisingly, the concept of "nature" or "natural" eludes simple, once-and-for-all definition. In his fine book *Humans in Nature: The World as We Find It and The World as We Create It*, Greg Kaebnick acknowledges the open-textured quality of these concepts and the reality that any definition offered will be endlessly contestable.[18] That's not a reason, however, to give up. He points out that a great many concepts we need and use regularly in thinking about morality have similarly eluded easy and precise definition, concepts such as "voluntary," "person," and "rational." In bioethics, after five decades of trying, we still lack a universally accepted definition of "death." That's the bad news. The good news is that despite lingering disagreement on defining death, we've been able to make progress on practical issues, for example, when it is permissible to recover organs from a newly dead body. Practical moral judgments, it turns out, don't have to be put off indefinitely until we have perfect agreement on the underlying concepts.

How we think about and regulate food provides an interesting parallel to doping in sport. Many people prefer their food to be "natural" or "organic," but a close examination of how we decide what counts as "natural" or "organic" shows a familiar definitional fuzziness. Despite that fuzziness, the United States Department of Agriculture has a policy on "natural" foods and a list of what to avoid in order for food to be labeled "organic."

"Organic" produce, for example, should involve no synthetic substances in its growing or handling—except that you can use certain copper-based insecticides; or hydrated lime, hydrogen peroxide, and potassium bicarbonate. And if you're growing pears or apples, you can use streptomycin to fight fire blight.

As you can see, the list is not conceptually pristine. It strives for minimal processing and additives but makes allowances for the realities of plant diseases and insects. But the list is useful, and it's far from arbitrary. Kaebnick writes: "In effect, these lists are attempts to work through a range of examples and, in so doing, to stipulate more precise understandings of what is inherently vague. The generation of these lists is not cut loose from the guidance of reason—it can be guided both by some general principles and by analogical reasoning from case to case . . . "[18 (p128)] The World Anti-Doping Agency's process for generating its annually revised list of prohibited substances and methods could be described in similar terms; Kaebnick uses the WADA list as another example of an imperfect, contestable, but useful and ultimately defensible way to make policy.

FAIRNESS, SAFETY AND MEANING

In the end, the three usual justifications offered for keeping performance-enhancing drugs out of sport—fairness, safety, and meaning—boil down to two: protecting athletes' health and preserving what's meaningful and valuable in sport. Safety—protecting athletes from harm—remains an important reason to deter doping, especially in light of the dynamic that drives athletes to match their competitors' use and the inevitability that PEDs will spread far beyond the privileged few elite athletes able to command expert medical management. Fairness becomes relevant to doping once we've decided doping should *not* be permitted. At that point, we have an obligation to provide non-doping athletes the reasonable assurance that doping won't overwhelm the competition. Fairness, though, doesn't tell us which performance-enhancing technologies to welcome and which to prohibit. For that, we need to understand what gives sport in general, and each particular sport, its values and meaning. Fortunately, the history of sport and the deep knowledge and commitment of those who play and understand it provide ample resources to inform those difficult judgments.

OTHER SPHERES

Understanding what to look for in the ethics of performance-enhancing technologies in sport offers a starting point for thinking about the place of technologies in other spheres of human life. Begin with the lived experience of people faced with decisions about using them. For sport, appreciating its inherent, relentlessly competitive structure is key. "Solutions" that fail to grasp how athletes' lives are shaped by that dynamic aren't likely to work. A "harm reduction" program can help people addicted to opiates who transmit disease through shared needles; it likely will fail abysmally for athletes looking for competitive advantages and determined not to surrender an edge.

As we seek insights into the ethics of enhancement in other realms of life, we should begin with attention to the realities and forces that shape people's interactions in each realm. Then we need to pay thoughtful attention to people's experiences. With a solid grasp of the realities of that particular realm, we can ask what values and meanings people seek there. Sport may be a relatively easy subject. Unlike many other spheres of human life, it's often called upon to be explicit about its values and meanings. When sport does its job well, it accepts or rejects innovations according to the values and meanings at its core. The task will be more difficult in spheres of life in which values and meanings are vague or contested. Let's briefly consider three important spheres: work, education, and love. I have more questions than answers.

WORK

On their first day as new associates at the prestigious white-shoe law firm Harass and Devour, the managing partner addresses the dozen attorneys who've just joined the firm. She lays out her expectation that they will bill many, many hours, working long days and into the night. She takes care to note that Harass and Devour would never, never *demand* that its employees take modafinil or other drugs that allow a person to keep working despite the overwhelming urge to sleep. But, she adds, there will always be an ample supply available in the pantry. At the end of a probationary period, three of the associates will be made partners; the other nine will have to look for work elsewhere. And she shall be watching your work very, very closely . . .

Workplaces that stress competition and maximum performance share some dynamics with competitive sport. Pressure to excel can push people to use drugs they believe enhance their ability to do the job. But there are important differences as well. In sport, performance is judged against both contemporary competitors and historical records. Athletes are not otherwise adding directly to the store of goods and services in the economy. And not all employers demand relentless productivity or pit their employees directly against one another—though some do. Employers' power over workers is another fundamental reality, as is the need for income and the satisfaction many people find in their work. All these factors have to be taken into account.

Economic, political, and social context are vital to understanding the ethics of enhancement for work, along with the role that work plays in individuals' identity and dignity. What are the principal values and meanings in this realm? What does it mean to have work? Are there values that reach across different types of work from poorly paid menial labor to well-compensated knowledge workers? From migrant farm workers to teachers to investment bankers? I can imagine possible values: the opportunity to demonstrate one's competence; taking pleasure in a task well done; satisfaction in giving a full day's effort; the camaraderie of shared labor and common purpose. What impact would biomedical performance enhancements have on those values and meanings? On workers' well-being and their possibilities for flourishing?

EDUCATION

Taking a drug to focus or to stave off fatigue may or may not be common in law firms, but pharmaceutical cognitive enhancement appears to be particularly popular in colleges and universities. In 2008, the journal *Nature* reported an online poll with 1,400 responses from sixty countries. The poll's design makes it impossible to generalize beyond the self-selected group of respondents, but the results were eye-catching. Asked about three kinds of drugs—methylphenidate (Ritalin), modafinil (Provigil), and beta blockers (to reduce anxiety)—one-fifth of the respondents reported using one or more of the drugs to improve focus, concentration, or memory, rather than for medical reasons. About half of those who used the drugs for nonmedical reasons reported side effects, including jitteriness, anxiety, headaches, and sleeplessness. The side effects were unpleasant enough to cause some people to stop.

The discussion around ethics was particularly interesting. Four out of five respondents said that healthy adults should be free to take the drugs if they wanted—a classic libertarian response. When it came to children younger than sixteen, though, the message was mixed. Respondents overwhelmingly supported restricting children's access to the drugs; but a third of them worried that they would be pressured to put their kids on drugs if their children's peers were using them. Why? They were fearful their children otherwise would be at a competitive disadvantage. The echoes of PEDs in sport are unmistakable.[19]

The scientific evidence on cognitive-enhancing drugs is mixed. There's some evidence they have a small to modest benefit for some people, but not reliably for everyone. More worrisome than short-term side effects is the possibility of long-term changes in the brain from chronic use. The younger the person using the drugs, the greater the concern about irreversible alterations in sensitive, still-developing brains.[20]

What do we value most in higher education? Suppose a dose of Ritalin boosted your ability to cram for an exam but had no impact on your long-term recollection of important facts. The higher test score would put pressure on your fellow test-takers to do the same, but what would it tell us about how well you understand what you've memorized or how creatively you could use it later?

The lure of the quick fix—the pill that solves an important problem in life—is understandable. Research often finds less dramatic effects in real-life settings than in labs. Then there's the likelihood of unwanted consequences: Biomedical enhancements at work and in education likely will have effects beyond those you seek. Would the distortions they might cause in judgment and common sense, mood or reasoning skills have any negative impact on your life or your faith in your own abilities?

LOVE

Finally, love. And voles. Specifically, prairie voles, who are known to be monogamous and eager to defend their families, and the closely related montane voles, who seem happy to mate with any partner and disinterested in defending the home front. Prairie voles have receptors for a pair of hormones in areas of the brain linked to reward and addiction. Oxytocin is associated with pair bonding; vasopressin, with territoriality. Montane voles don't have the same pattern of receptors in their brains. Scientists are finding that oxytocin also has an impact on how humans respond to possible partners, but the results so far are complicated.[21] That hasn't prevented people from speculating on the use of something such as inhaled oxytocin to promote marital fidelity.

In an article charmingly titled "The Medicalization of Love," the authors point out a variety of ways we can give our bodies a surge of oxytocin, including going to couples therapy, getting a massage, or having sex. If a couple pursued any or all of these activities in order to improve their relationship, we'd have no objection. So, the authors ask, "That being the case . . . it is not at all clear that the exogenous modification of that same brain chemistry—especially in a similar behavioral context, yet through the use of an oxytocin nasal spray . . . would introduce a special moral problem."[22 (p330-331)]

Some people might object that a quick squirt up the nose is not an authentic way to deepen your bond with the one you love. The article's authors hint that authenticity may be overrated: " . . . within the hierarchy of values for a particular couple, a happy or well-functioning relationship may be more important than an abstract notion of authenticity. It would seem reasonable to argue that couples should be able to pursue their highest values by whatever (legal) means . . ."[22 (p331)] And if those values include monogamy, a squirt is as good as a . . . well, any of those alternative ways to get oxytocin to the brain.

We've come full circle, I think. The problem with blood doping, EPO, or other performance-enhancing drugs for athletes was that it disrupted the connection between talent and dedication on the one hand and improved performance on the other. Is there meaning and value in caressing someone you love, listening attentively, or making love for which a spurt from a plastic squeeze bottle of oxytocin is not an adequate substitute? It depends, I suppose, on what you believe matters in your most important, enduring, loving relationships. In the ethics of enhancement, it always comes down to values and meaning.

"THE TISSUE-THIN DIFFERENCE . . ."

John Updike captured the essence of baseball's grandeur in his *New Yorker* essay on Ted Williams's last game at Fenway Park on 28 September 1960. (His essay carries one of the best titles ever: "Hub Fans Bid Kid Adieu." Say that aloud.) Williams's enormous pride and his dedication to the craft of hitting a baseball did not guarantee a warm relationship with his fans. Updike offers this description of baseball's nature and Williams's accomplishments:

> It may be that, compared to managers' dreams such as Joe DiMaggio and the always helpful Stan Musial, Williams is an icy star. But of all team sports, baseball, with its graceful intermittences of action, its immense and tranquil field sparsely settled with poised men in white, its dispassionate mathematics, seems to me best suited to accommodate, and be ornamented by, a loner. It is an essentially lonely game. No other player visible to my generation has concentrated within himself so much of the sport's poignance, has so assiduously refined his natural skills, has so constantly brought to the plate that intensity of competence that crowds the throat with joy.[23]

The fundamental loneliness of baseball, Williams's remarkable talents, his unexcelled dedication to perfecting them, and his intense pride in his work: all captured economically in a single paragraph: The great writer on the great hitter. Did Updike perhaps see in Williams an echo of his life as a writer? Loneliness, talent, dedication, pride, intensity: These traits describe them both. We find here both a brilliant account of why we care about baseball, what we value in it, and of the relationship of those elements of value to our lives beyond sport. Updike describes it as "the tissue-thin difference between a thing done well and a thing done ill." Caring enough to do your best, give the full measure of effort, when few will notice and when the impact of your striving on the longer arc of a season or a life is impossible to discern.

In his last at-bat, during the eighth inning of the final home game for his Boston Red Sox, after taking the first pitch as a ball,

Williams swung at the next pitch—and missed. The third pitch arrived. Williams's devotion to his art yielded one last fruit: The ball sailed over the center-field fence—a home run, the five hundred and twenty-first of a brilliant career, interrupted by injury and war, yet triumphant in its skill, dedication, and perseverance. Here is Updike's description of what followed: "Though we thumped, wept, and chanted 'We want Ted' for minutes after he hid in the dugout, he did not come back. Our noise for some seconds passed beyond excitement into a kind of immense open anguish, a wailing, a cry to be saved. But immortality is nontransferable. The papers said that the other players, and even the umpires on the field, begged him to come out and acknowledge us in some way, but he never had and did not now. Gods do not answer letters."

Why should a worldly, sophisticated, immensely perceptive writer such as John Updike care about an aging ballplayer? There must be more to sport than merely spectacle and entertainment. I'm thinking again of Bill Bradley's description of his joy in the flow of a basketball game as the talents of individuals merged into an extraordinary team: "In my Knicks days, there was no feeling comparable to the one I got when the team's game came together—those nights when five guys moved as one. The moment was one of beautiful isolation, the result of the correct blending of human forces at the proper time and to the exact degree. With my team, before the crowd, against our opponents, it was almost as if this were my private world and no one else could sense the inexorable rightness of the moment." There were also times of exaltation: "In plenty of games, I played simply for the joy of it, shooting and passing without thinking about points. I forgot the score, and sometimes I would go through a whole quarter without looking at the scoreboard."[24]

I suspect that many people, at all levels of talent and skill, have had glimpses in their sport of what Bill Bradley describes. I know I have, however few and fleeting. If so, you've experienced what Updike called "the tissue-thin difference between a thing done well and a thing done ill." The question before us is on what side of that line doping belongs.

NOTES

1. Murray T, Murray P. Rawls, Sports, and liberal legitimacy. In Kaebnick GE, editor. *The Ideal of Nature: Debates about Biotechnology and the Environment*. Baltimore: Johns Hopkins University Press; 2011. p. 179–199.
2. Rawls J. *Political Liberalism*. Expanded edition. New York: Columbia University Press; 2005. 525 p.
3. Walzer M. *Spheres of Justice: a Defense of Pluralism and Equality*. New York: Basic Books; 1983. 366 p.
4. Franke WW, Berendonk B. Hormonal doping and androgenization of athletes: A secret program of the German Democratic Republic government. *Clin Chem*. 1997;43(7):1262–1279.
5. Hoberman J. How drug testing fails: The politics of doping control. In: Wilson W, Derse E, editors. *Doping in Elite Sport: The Politics of Drugs in the Olympic Movement*. New York: Human Kinetics; 2001. p. 241–270.
6. Panel of the IAAF Ethics Commission. Ethics Commission Decision – VB, AM, GD, PMD - Decision No 02/2016. 2016. Available from: https://www.iaafethicsboard.org/decisions.
7. Pound RW, McLaren RH, Younger G. Independent Commission Report #1 World Anti-Doping Agency [Internet]. 2015 Nov 19. Available from: https://www.wada-ama.org/en/resources/world-anti-doping-program/independent-commission-report-1.
8. Pound RW, McLaren RH, Younger G. WADA Independent Commission Report part 2 [Internet]. 2016. Available from: https://www.wada-ama.org/sites/default/files/resources/files/wada_independent_commission_report_2_2016_en_rev.pdf.
9. McLaren RH. The Independent Person Report [Internet]. 2016 Jul 16. Available from: https://www.wada-ama.org/sites/default/files/resources/files/20160718_ip_report_newfinal.pdf.

10. McLaren RH. The Independent Person 2nd Report [Internet]. World Anti-Doping Agency; 2016 Dec 9 [cited 2017 Jan 3]. Available from: https://www.wada-ama.org/sites/default/files/resources/files/mclaren_report_part_ii_2.pdf.

11. Widdicombe L. The end of food. *The New Yorker* [Internet]. 2014 May 12 [cited 2016 Aug 3]. Available from: http://www.newyorker.com/magazine/2014/05/12/the-end-of-food.

12. Loland S. The ethics of performance-enhancing technology in sport. *J Philos Sport.* 2009;36(2):152–161.

13. Savulesu J, Foddy B, Clayton M. Why we should allow performance enhancing drugs in sport. *Br J Sports Med.* 2004 Dec;38(6):666–674.

14. Bostrom N. Letter from Utopia. *Stud Ethics Law Technol.* 2008;2(1):1–7.

15. McNamee MJ, Edwards SD. Transhumanism, medical technology and slippery slopes. *J Med Ethics.* 2006;32(9):513–518.

16. Miah A. Enhanced athletes? It's only natural [Internet]. *Washington Post.* 2008 Aug 3 [cited 2016 Dec 28]. Available from: http://www.washingtonpost.com/wp-dyn/content/article/2008/08/01/AR2008080103060.html.

17. Todd J, Todd T. Reflections on the "parallel federation solution" to the problem of drug use in sport: The cautionary tale of powerlifting. In T. H. Murray, K. J. Maschke, and A. A. Wasunna, eds. *Performance-Enhancing Technologies in Sports: Ethical, Conceptual, and Scientific Issues.* Baltimore: Johns Hopkins University Press; 2009. p. 44–80.

18. Kaebnick GE. *Humans in Nature: The World as We Find It and the World as We Create It.* New York: Oxford University Press; 2013. 224 p.

19. Maher B. Poll results: Look who's doping. *Nature.* 2008 Apr 9;452(7188):674–675.

20. Sahakian BJ, Morein-Zamir S. Pharmacological cognitive enhancement: Treatment of neuropsychiatric disorders and lifestyle use by healthy people. *Lancet Psychiatry.* 2015;2(4):357–362.

21. Tucker A. What can rodents tell us about why humans love? *Smithsonian* [Internet]. 2014 Feb [cited 2016 Aug 5]. Available from: http://www.smithsonianmag.com/science-nature/what-can-rodents-tell-us-about-why-humans-love-180949441/.

22. Earp BD, Sandberg A, Savulescu J. The medicalization of love. *Cambridge Q Health Ethics.* 2015 Jul;24(3):323–336.

23. Updike J. Hub fans bid kid adieu [Internet]. *The New Yorker.* 1960 Oct 22 [cited 2016 Dec 28]. Available from: http://www.newyorker.com/magazine/1960/10/22/hub-fans-bid-kid-adieu.

24. Bradley B. *Values of the Game.* New York: Broadway; 2000. 96 p.

BIBLIOGRAPHY

Ahmad C.S., Grantham W.J., and Greiwe R.M. 2012. Public perceptions of Tommy John surgery. *The Physician and Sports Medicine* 40(2):64–72.

Amdur N. 1978. Mounting drug use afflicts world sports. *New York Times.* 1978 Nov 20. Available from: http://www.nytimes.com/1978/11/20/archives/mounting-drug-use-afflicts-world-sports-drug-epidemic-afflicts.html.

Aristotle. 1941. *Politics.* New York: Random House.

Associated Press. Greek federation suspends Halkia two years for doping. *ESPN.com.* 2008 Nov 27. Available from: http://espn.go.com/olympics/trackandfield/news/story?id=3730257.

A.T. Kearney, LLC. Winning in the business of sport. 2014. Available from: https://www.atkearney.com/documents/10192/5258876/Winning+in+the+Business+of+Sports.pdf/ed85b644-7633-469d-8f7a-99e4a50aadc8.

Austin S. 2014. I quit cycling because of the drugs. Now I am Lance Armstrong's best riding buddy. *The Telegraph.* 2014 Jan 9. Available from: http://www.telegraph.co.uk/sport/othersports/cycling/10562181/I-quit-cycling-because-of-the-drugs.-Now-I-am-Lance-Armstrongs-best-riding-buddy.html.

Barrow J.D. 2012. Why ban full-body Olympics swimsuits? A scientist explains polyurethane. *The Daily Beast.* 2012 Jul 25. Available from: http://www.thedailybeast.com/articles/2012/07/25/why-ban-full-body-olympics-swimsuits-a-scientist-explains-polyurethane.html.

BBC News. 1998. Drugs stance stirs outrage. *BBC.* Available from: http://news.bbc.co.uk/2/hi/sport/140315.stm.

BBC News. 2016. Rio Paralympics 2016: Classification is "bedrock" of sport says BPA chief. *BBC Sport.* Available from: http://www.bbc.com/sport/disability-sport/37286362.

Bell S. 2015. What we've missed about Tommy John surgery. *ESPN.com.* 2015 Apr 9. Available from: http://espn.go.com/mlb/story/_/id/12648769.

Berg S. 2009. 1936 Berlin Olympics: How Dora the man competed in the woman's high jump. *Der Spiegel Online.* 2009 Sept 15. Available from: http://www.spiegel.de/international/germany/1936-berlin-olympics-how-dora-the-man-competed-in-the-woman-s-high-jump-a-649104.html.

Bermon S., et al. 2014. Serum androgen levels in elite female athletes. *The Journal of Clinical Endocrinology & Metabolism* 99(11):4328–4335.

Blauwet C.A., Benjamin-Laing H., Stomphorst J., Van de Vliet P., Pit-Grosheide P., and Willick S.E. 2013. Testing for boosting at the Paralympic games: Policies, results and future directions. *British Journal of Sports Medicine* 47(13):832–837.

Bostrom N. 2008. Letter from Utopia. *Studies in Ethics, Law, and Technology* 2(1, article 6):1–7.

Bradley B. 2000. *Values of the Game.* New York: Broadway.

Brio D.L. 1990. Of MDs and muscles: Lessons from two "retired steroid doctors." *JAMA: The Journal of the American Medical Association* 263(12):1697–1705.

Brooks M.A. 2011. Genetic testing and youth sports. *JAMA: The Journal of the American Medical Association* 305(10):1033–1034.

Bull A. 2016. Caster Semenya wins gold but faces more scrutiny as IAAF press case. *The Guardian.* 2016 Aug 21. Available from: https://www.theguardian.com/sport/2016/aug/21/caster-semenya-wins-gold-but-faces-scrutiny.

Burke M.D., and Roberts T.J. 1997. Drugs in sport: An issue of morality or sentimentality. *Journal of the Philosophy of Sport* 24(1):99–113.

Callow J. 2010. Caster Semenya faces growing backlash after competitors have their say. *The Guardian.* 2010 Aug 23. Available from: https://www.theguardian.com/sport/2010/aug/23/caster-semenya-backlash-jemma-simpson.

Carlson A. 1991. When is a woman not a woman? For 24 years Maria Patino thought she was female. Then she failed the sex test. *Women's Sport & Fitness* 1991 Mar:24–29.

de la Chapelle A, Träskelin A.L., and Juvonen E. 1993. Truncated erythropoietin receptor causes dominantly inherited benign human erythrocytosis. *Proceedings of the National Academy of Sciences of the United States of America* 90(10):4495–4499.

Coletta A. 2016. Speedskater is poised to upend rule of sports' highest court. *New York Times.* 2016 Feb 11. Available from: http://www.nytimes.com/

2016/02/12/sports/skater-challenges-supremacy-of-court-of-arbitra-tion-for-sport.html.

Collier R. 2008. Most Paralympians inspire, but others cheat. *CMAJ: Canadian Medical Association Journal* 179(6):524.

Conte S.A., Fleisig G.S., Dines J.S., Wilk K.E., Aune K.T., Patterson-Flynn N., et al. Prevalence of ulnar collateral ligament surgery in professional baseball players. *American Journal of Sports Medicine.* 2015 Jul 1;43(7):1764–1769.

Court of Arbitration for Sport. 2015. *Interim Arbitral Award Dutee Chand v. AFI & IAAF.* Available from: http://www.tas-cas.org/fileadmin/user_upload/award_internet.pdf.

Coyle D., and Hamilton T. 2012. *The Secret Race: Inside the Hidden World of the Tour de France: Doping, Cover-ups, and Winning at All Costs.* New York: Bantam.

Crouse K. 2009. Faster racing suits may soon be banned from competition. *New York Times.* 2009 May 18. Available from: http://www.nytimes.com/2009/05/18/sports/othersports/18swim.html.

Earp B.D., Sandberg A., and Savulescu J. 2015. The medicalization of love. *Cambridge Quarterly of Healthcare Ethics* 24(3):323–336.

Elsas L.J., et al. 2000. Gender verification of female athletes. *Genetics in Medicine* 2(4):249–254.

Epstein D. 2014. *The Sports Gene: Inside the Science of Extraordinary Athletic Performance.* New York: Current.

Federation of Gay Games. 2017. Gender in sport. Available from: https://gaygames.org/wp/sport/sports-policiesd/gender/.

Fénichel P. et al. 2013. Molecular diagnosis of 5α-reductase deficiency in 4 elite young female athletes through hormonal screening for hyperandrogenism. *The Journal of Clinical Endocrinology & Metabolism* 98(6):E1055–E1059.

Fost N. 1986. Banning drugs in sports: A skeptical view. *The Hastings Center Report* 16(4):5–10.

Franke W.W., and B. Berendonk. 1997. Hormonal doping and androgeniza-tion of athletes: A secret program of the German Democratic Republic government. *Clinical Chemistry* 43(7):1262–1279.

Ganslen RV. 1973. *Mechanics of the Pole Vault.* St. Louis, MO: John Swift Co.

Genel, M., and Ljungqvist A. 2005. Gender verification of female athletes. *Lancet* 366(Medicine and Sport):S41.

Gilbert B. 1969. Problems in a turned-on world. *Sports Illustrated.* 1969 Jun 23.

Gladwell M. 2013. Man And superman. *The New Yorker.* 2013 Sept 9. Available from: http://www.newyorker.com/magazine/2013/09/09/man-and-superman.

Glanville D. 2010. Desperately seeking blank. *The Pennsylvania Gazette.* 2010 Jul/Aug. Available from: http://www.upenn.edu/gazette/0710/fea-ture2_1.html.

Gold J.R., and Gold M.M. 2007. Access for all: The rise of the Paralympic Games. *The Journal of the Royal Society for the Promotion of Health* 127(3):133–141.

Govender P. 2010. South African Semenya cleared to return. *Reuters*. Available from: http://www.reuters.com/article/us-athletics-semenya-idUSTRE6652M320100706.

Gundersen K. 2016. Muscle memory and a new cellular model for muscle atrophy and hypertrophy. *Journal of Experimental Biology* 219(2):235–242.

Halberstam D. 2009. *The Breaks of the Game*. New York: Hyperion.

Hanstad D.V., Skille E.Å., and Thurston M. 2009. Elite athletes' perspectives on providing whereabouts information: A survey of athletes in the Norwegian registered testing pool. *Sport and Society* 6(1):30–46.

Hoberman J. 2001. How drug testing fails: the politics of doping control. In W. Wilson & E. Derse, eds. *Doping in Elite Sport: The Politics of Drugs in the Olympic Movement*. New York: Human Kinetics, 241–270.

Hoberman J. 2002. Sports physicians and the doping crisis in elite sport. *Clinical Journal of Sport Medicine* 12(4):203–208.

Hoberman J. 2005. *Testosterone Dreams: Rejuvenation, Aphrodisia, Doping*. Berkeley: University of California Press.

Hoberman J. 2012. Sports physicians and doping: Medical ethics and elite performance. In Malcolm D. and Safai, P., eds. *The Social Organization of Sports Medicine: Critical Socio-Cultural Perspectives*. London and New York: Routledge, 247–264.

Hobson W. 2016. Olympic executives cash in on a "Movement" that keeps athletes poor. *The Washington Post*. 2016 July 30. Available from: https://www.washingtonpost.com/sports/olympics/olympic-executives-cash-in-on-a-movement-that-keeps-athletes-poor/2016/07/30/ed18c206-5346-11e6-88eb-7dda4e2f2aec_story.html.

Howe D. 2008. *The Cultural Politics of the Paralympic Movement: Through an Anthropological Lens*. London: Routledge.

Ingle S. 2016. British athletes demand stronger action from WADA on drug cheats. *The Guardian*. 2016 Jun 13. Available from: https://www.theguardian.com/sport/2016/jun/13/british-athletes-letter-world-anti-doping-agency-drug-cheats.

International Olympic Committee. 2016. Olympic Charter. Available from: https://stillmed.olympic.org/media/Document%20Library/OlympicOrg/General/EN-Olympic-Charter.pdf.

International Paralympic Committee. Historical Results. Available from: https://www.paralympic.org/results/historical.

International Paralympic Committee. 2016. International Paralympic Committee Athletics Rules and Regulations 2016–2017. Jan 2016.

Available from: https://www.paralympic.org/sites/default/files/document/160126174701371_2016_01_26+IPC+Athletics+Rules+and+Regulations_A4_Final.pdf.

International Skating Union. 2014. International Skating Union Special Reguations & Technical Rules Single & Pair Skating. Available from: http://static.isu.org/media/166717/2014-special-regulation-sandp-and-ice-dance-and-technical-rules-sandp-and-id_14-09-16.pdf.

IOC. 2015. IOC consensus meeting on sex reassignment and hyperandrogenism November 2015. Available from: http://www.triathlon.org/uploads/docs/6.b_2015.11_IOC_consensus_meeting_on_sex_reassignment_and_hyperandrogenism-ENG.pdf.

Johnson J., Butryn T., and Masucci M. 2013. A focus group analysis of the US and Canadian female triathletes' knowledge of doping. *Sport in Society* 16(5):654–671.

Kaebnick G.E. 2013. *Humans in Nature: The World As We Find It and the World As We Create It*. New York: Oxford University Press.

Karkazis K. et al. 2012. Out of bounds? A critique of the new policies on hyperandrogenism in elite female athletes. *The American Journal of Bioethics* 12(7):3–16.

Kayser B., Mauron A., and Miah A. 2005. Viewpoint: Legalisation of performance-enhancing drugs. *Lancet*, 366 Suppl:S21.

Kayser B., Mauron A., and Miah A. 2007. Current anti-doping policy: A critical appraisal. *BMC Medical Ethics* 8(2):1–10.

Kayser B., and Smith A.C.T. 2008. Globalisation of anti-doping: The reverse side of the medal. *British Medical Journal* 337(7661):85–87.

Kreft L. 2011. Elite sportspersons and commodity control: Anti-doping as quality assurance. *International Journal of Sport Policy and Politics* Jul;3(2):151–161.

Lodewijkx H.F.M., Brouwe B., Kuipers H., and Hezewijk R. van. 2013. Overestimated effect of EPO administration on aerobic exercise capacity: A meta-analysis. *American Journal of Sports Science and Medicine* 1(2):17–27.

Loland S. 2009. The ethics of performance-enhancing technology in sport. *Journal of the Philosophy of Sport* 36(2):152–161.

Loland S., and Hoppeler H. 2012. Justifying anti-doping: The fair opportunity principle and the biology of performance enhancement. *European Journal of Sport Science* 12(4):347–353.

Loland S., and Murray T.H. 2007. The ethics of the use of technologically constructed high-altitude environments to enhance performances in sport. *Scandinavian Journal of Medicine & Science in Sports* 17(3):193–193.

Maennig W. 2014. Inefficiency of the anti-doping system: Cost reduction proposals. *Substance Use & Misuse* 49(9):1201–1205.

Maher B. 2008. Poll results: Look who's doping. *Nature* 452(7188): 674–675.

Martínez-Patiño M.J. 2005. Personal account: A woman tried and tested. Special Issue: Medicine and Sport. *The Lancet* 9503:S38.

Martínez-Patiño M.J. 2016. Maria Jose Martinez Patiño Personal Communication.

McDonald H. 2015. Ireland passes law allowing trans people to choose their legal gender. *The Guardian*. 2015 Jul 16. Available from: http://www.theguardian.com/world/2015/jul/16/ireland-transgender-law-gender-recognition-bill-passed.

McGee B. 2012. How dopers stole the best years of my career. *Sidney Morning Herald*. 2012 Oct 27. Available from: http://www.smh.com.au/sport/cycling/how-dopers-stole-the-best-years-of-my-career-20121026-28aif.html.

McLaren R.H. 2016a. The Independent Person 2nd Report. 2016 Dec 9. Available from: https://www.wada-ama.org/sites/default/files/resources/files/mclaren_report_part_ii_2.pdf.

McLaren R.H. 2016b. The Independent Person Report. Jul 16. Available from: https://www.wada-ama.org/sites/default/files/resources/files/20160718_ip_report_newfinal.pdf.

McNamee M.J., and Edwards S.D. 2006. Transhumanism, medical technology, and slippery slopes. *Journal of Medical Ethics* 32(9):513–518.

Mehlman M. 2009. Genetic enhancement in sport: Ethical, legal and policy concerns. In T. H. Murray, K. J. Maschke, and A. A. Wasunna, eds. *Performance-Enhancing Technologies in Sports: Ethical, Conceptual, and Scientific Issues*. Baltimore: Johns Hopkins University Press, 205–224.

Miah A. 2008. Enhanced athletes? It's only natural. *Washington Post*. 2008 Aug 3. Available from: http://www.washingtonpost.com/wp-dyn/content/article/2008/08/01/AR2008080103060.html.

Murray T., and Murray P. 2011. Rawls, sports, and liberal legitimacy. In Kaebnick, GE, editor. *The Ideal of Nature: Debates about Biotechnology and the Environment*. Baltimore: Johns Hopkins University Press, 179–199.

Murray T.H. 1983. The coercive power of drugs in sports. *The Hastings Center Report* 13(4):24–30.

Murray T.H. 2014. Stirring the simmering "designer baby" pot. *Science* 343(6176):1208–1210.

National Federation of State High School Associations, 2015–16 High School Athletics Participation Survey. Available from: http://www.nfhs.org/ParticipationStatistics/PDF/2015-16_Sports_Participation_Survey.pdf.

O'Connor L.M., and Vozenilek J.A. 2011. Is it the athlete or the equipment? An analysis of the top swim performances from 1990 to 2010. *Journal of Strength and Conditioning Research/National Strength & Conditioning Association* 25(12):3239–3241.

Overbye M., and Wagner U. 2013. Experiences, attitudes and trust: An inquiry into elite athletes' perception of the whereabouts reporting system. *International Journal of Sport Policy and Politics* 6(3):1–22

Panel of the IAAF Ethics Commission. 2016. Ethics Commission Decision – VB, AM, GD, PMD—Decision No 02/2016.pdf. Available from: https://www.iaafethicsboard.org/decisions.

Peterson R. 1992. *Only the Ball Was White: A History of Legendary Black Players and All-Black Professional Teams.* Oxford: Oxford University Press, 1992.

Pound R.W., McLaren R.H., and Younger G. 2015. Independent Commission Report #1 World Anti-Doping Agency. Available from: https://www.wada-ama.org/en/resources/world-anti-doping-program/independent-commission-report-1.

Pound R.W., McLaren R.H., and Younger G. 2016. WADA Independent Commission Report part 2. Available from: https://www.wada-ama.org/sites/default/files/resources/files/wada_independent_commission_report_2_2016_en_rev.pdf.

pwc.com/sports outlook. 2011. Changing the game: Outlook for the global sports market to 2015. 2011 Dec. Available from: http://www.pwc.com/gx/en/hospitality-leisure/pdf/changing-the-game-outlook-for-the-global-sports-market-to-2015.pdf.

Rawls J. 1981. Letter to Owen Fiss. *The Boston Review.* 1981. Available from: http://bostonreview.net/rawls-the-best-of-all-games.

Rawls J. 1999. *A Theory of Justice.* Revised edition. Cambridge, MA: Belknap.

Rawls J. 2005. *Political Liberalism* Expanded edition. New York: Columbia University Press.

Reeser J.C. 2005. Gender identity and sport: Is the playing field level? *British Journal of Sports Medicine* 39(10):695–699.

Rhodan M. 2014. Olympic committee adds anti-discrimination clause for host cities. *Time.* 2014 Sept 24. Available from: http://time.com/3427596/olympic-committee-host-discrimination/.

Ruiz R.R., and Schwirtz M. 2016. Russian insider says state-run doping fueled Olympic gold. *New York Times.* 2016 May 12. Available from: http://www.nytimes.com/2016/05/13/sports/russia-doping-sochi-olympics-2014.html.

Sahakian B.J., and Morein-Zamir S. 2015. Pharmacological cognitive enhancement: Treatment of neuropsychiatric disorders and lifestyle use by healthy people. *The Lancet Psychiatry* 2(4):357–362.

Sakamoto H. et al. 1988. Femininity control at the XXth Universiade in Kobe, Japan. *International Journal of Sports Medicine* 9(3):193–195.

Sandel M.J. 2007. *The Case against Perfection: Ethics in the Age of Genetic Engineering*. Cambridge, MA: Belknap.

Savulescu J. 2016. Doping scandals, Rio, and the future of human enhancement: Editorial. *Bioethics* 30(5):300–303.

Savulescu J., and Foddy B. 2011. Le Tour and failure of zero tolerance: Time to relax doping controls. In Savulescu J., ter Meulen R., and Kahane G., editors. *Enhancing Human Capacities*. Oxford: Wiley Blackwell, 304–312.

Savulescu J., Foddy B., and Clayton M. 2004. Why we should allow performance enhancing drugs in sport. *British Journal of Sports Medicine* 38(6):666–674.

Sengupta R. 2014. Why Dutee Chand can change sports. *Live Mint*. Available from: http://www.livemint.com/Leisure/9P3jbOG2G0ppTVB7Xvwj0K/Why-Dutee-Chand-can-change-sports.html.

Siebenmann C., Robach P., Jacobs R.A., Rasmussen P., Nordsborg N., Diaz V., et al. 2011. "Live high–train low" using normobaric hypoxia: A double-blinded, placebo-controlled study. *Journal of Applied Physiology* 112(1):106–117.

Silverman I. 2016. The IPC's statement related to intentional misrepresentation. *SwimSwam*. 2016 Aug 12. Available from: https://swimswam.com/ipcs-statement-related-intentional-misrepresentation/.

Simon R.L. 2016. *The Ethics of Sport: What Everyone Needs to Know*. New York: Oxford University Press.

Sinex J.A., and Chapman R.F. 2015. Hypoxic training methods for improving endurance exercise performance. *Journal of Sport and Health Science* 4(4):325–332.

Sjoqvist F., Garle M., and Rane A. 2008. Use of doping agents, particularly anabolic steroids, in sports and society. *Lancet* 371(9627):1872–1882.

Smith D. 2009. Report claims 800m world champion Caster Semenya is a hermaphrodite. 2009 Sept 10. *The Guardian*. Available from: https://www.theguardian.com/sport/2009/sep/10/caster-semenya-hermaphrodite-iaaf-test.

Stokes S. 2013. Michael Rasmussen retires and admits doping over a fourteen year timeframe. *Velonation*. 2013 Jan 31. Available from: http://www.velonation.com/News/ID/13829/Michael-Rasmussen-retires-and-admits-doping-over-a-fourteen-year-timeframe.aspx.

Swarbrick S. 2011. Cyclist David Millar tells of his battle with drugs. *The Herald (Scotland)*. 13th Sept 2011. Available from: http://www.herald-scotland.com/life_style/13041664.Cyclist_David_Millar_tells_of_his_battle_with_drugs/.

Tamburrini C.M. 2007. What's wrong with genetic inequality? The impact of genetic technology on elite sports and society. *Sport, Ethics and Philosophy* 1(2):229–238.

Tännsjö T. 2005. Hypoxic air machines: Commentary. *Journal of Medical Ethics* 31(2):113–113.

Todd J., and Todd T. 2009. Reflections on the "parallel federation solution" to the problem of drug use in sport: The cautionary tale of powerlifting. In T. H. Murray, K. J. Maschke, and A. A. Wasunna, eds. *Performance-Enhancing Technologies in Sports: Ethical, Conceptual, and Scientific Issues.* Baltimore: Johns Hopkins University Press, 44–80.

Tremlett G. 2004. The cheats. *The Guardian.* 2004 Sept 15. Available from: https://www.theguardian.com/sport/2004/sep/16/gilestremlett. features11.

Tucker A. 2014. What can rodents tell us about why humans love? *Smithsonian.* Available from: http://www.smithsonianmag.com/science-nature/ what-can-rodents-tell-us-about-why-humans-love-180949441/.

Tweedy, S.M., 2009. Discussion Paper—Changing the eligibility criterion for unilateral upper limb amputation in IPC Athletics, Presented at IPC Athletics Summit, 2009, Bonn Germany.

Tweedy S.M., and Vanlandewijck Y.C. 2009. International Paralympic Committee position stand: Background and scientific principles of classification in Paralympic sport. *British Journal of Sports Medicine* 45(4):259–269. Available from: http://www.ncbi.nlm.nih.gov/pubmed/ 19850575.

Tweedy S.M., Williams G., and Bourke J. 2010. Selecting and modifying methods of manual muscle testing for classification in Paralympic sport. *European Journal of Adapted Physical Activity* 3(2):7–16.

Updike J. 1960. Hub fans bid kid adieu. *The New Yorker.* 1960 Oct 22. Available from: http://www.newyorker.com/magazine/1960/10/22/ hub-fans-bid-kid-adieu.

U.S. Anti-Doping Agency (USADA) (n.d.) U.S. Postal Service Pro Cycling Team Investigation. Available from: http://cyclinginvestigation.usada.org/.

US Food and Drug Administration. 2011. Press Announcements—FDA modifies dosing recommendations for erythropoiesis-stimulating agents. Available from: http://www.fda.gov/NewsEvents/Newsroom/ PressAnnouncements/ucm260670.htm.

Valkenburg D., de Hon O., and van Hilvoorde I. 2014. Doping control, providing whereabouts and the importance of privacy for elite athletes. *International Journal of Drug Policy* 25(2):212–218.

van Hilvoorde I., Vos R., and de Wert G. 2007. Flopping, klapping, and gene doping: Dichotomies between "natural" and "artificial" in elite sports. *Social Studies of Science* 37:173–200.

Vaughters J. 2012. How to get doping out of sport. *NYTimes.com.* 2012 Aug 8. Available from: http://www.nytimes.com/2012/08/12/opinion/sunday/how-to-get-doping-out-of-sports.html.

VeloNews. 2016. Van den Driessche banned six years for hidden motor. *VeloNews.com*. 2016 Apr 26. Available from: http://velonews.competitor.com/2016/04/news/van-den-driessche-banned-six-years-for-hidden-motor_403450.

Versteeg R. 2005. Arresting vaulting pole technology. *Vanderbilt Journal of Entertainment and Tech. Law* 8(1):93–117.

Vinton N. 2009. Former East German track coach Ekkart Arbeit caught up in Caster Semenya gender controversy. *NY Daily News*. Available from: http://www.nydailynews.com/sports/more-sports/east-german-track-coach-ekkart-arbeit-caught-caster-semenya-gender-controversy-article-1.397564.

Vonnegut K. 2008. *Welcome to the Monkey House*. Reprint edition. New York: Paw Prints.

Waddington I., and Smith A. 2000. *Sport, Health and Drugs: A Critical Sociological Perspective*. London and New York: Routledge.

Walzer M. 1983. *Spheres of Justice: a Defense of Pluralism and Equality*. New York: Basic Books.

Widdicombe L. 2014. The end of food. *The New Yorker*. 2014 May 12. Available from: http://www.newyorker.com/magazine/2014/05/12/the-end-of-food.

Wiedeman R. 2016. A full revolution: In the run-up to the Olympics, Simone Biles is transforming gymnastics. *The New Yorker*. 2016 May 30. Available from: http://www.newyorker.com/magazine/2016/05/30/simone-biles-is-the-best-gymnast-in-the-world.

Wilson J.M. et al. 2012. The effects of endurance, strength, and power training on muscle fiber type shifting. *Journal of Strength and Conditioning Research* 26(6):1724–1729.

INDEX